Malyhe Jalilvand

Application-Specific Broadband Antennas for Microwave Medical Imaging

Karlsruher Forschungsberichte
aus dem Institut für Hochfrequenztechnik und Elektronik

Herausgeber: Prof. Dr.-Ing. Thomas Zwick

Band 85

Eine Übersicht aller bisher in dieser Schriftenreihe erschienenen Bände finden Sie am Ende des Buches.

Application-Specific Broadband Antennas for Microwave Medical Imaging

by

Malyhe Jalilvand

Scientific Publishing

Dissertation, Karlsruher Institut für Technologie
KIT-Fakultät für Elektrotechnik und Informationstechnik

Tag der mündlichen Prüfung: 17. Oktober 2016
Referenten: Prof. Dr.-Ing. Thomas Zwick
Prof. Dr. rer. nat. Olaf Dössel

Impressum

KIT Scientific Publishing

Karlsruher Institut für Technologie (KIT)
KIT Scientific Publishing
Straße am Forum 2
D-76131 Karlsruhe

KIT Scientific Publishing is a registered trademark
of Karlsruhe Institute of Technology.
Reprint using the book cover is not allowed.

www.ksp.kit.edu

Print on Demand 2017 – Gedruckt auf FSC-zertifiziertem Papier

ISSN 1868-4696
ISBN 978-3-7315-0664-5
DOI 10.5445/KSP/1000069288

Editor's Preface

Medical diagnostics by means of microwaves is a growing research field worldwide since nearly 20 years. Although, such systems are unlikely to achieve the high performance of the existing technologies such as magnetic resonance imaging (MRI), computed tomography (CT) and ultrasound in general, the imaging systems based on electromagnetic waves can be an attractive extension to these existing systems. For one thing, the new systems could be significantly cheaper and more portable than MRI and CT, for another thing, they have an advantage over ultrasound as they can âseeâ through bones. A very interesting application could therefore be the identification and classification of stroke. First, the skull/cranial bones prevent the successful use of ultrasound and second, a very quick outpatient distinction between ischemic and hemorrhagic stroke is crucial for successful treatment.

Since microwave-based diagnostic systems could easily be implemented as compact and portable systems, this appears to be one of the most attractive areas of application of the new technology. However, there is a problem common to all microwave medical diagnostic applications: the relatively high signal attenuation in the tissues and the reflection of the waves from the surface of the body. An important approach to solving this problem is to place the antennas directly on the body to avoid the high reflection at the interface between air and tissue. At the same time, this method promises reduced antenna size, which is essential for imaging systems, where a maximum number of systems, i.e. antennas are beneficial. Furthermore, the antennas are an ultimate part of the imaging system and therefore have a huge impact on the resulting image quality.

In her work, Ms. Jalilvand provided important scientific fundamentals to specific antennas for medical microwave diagnostics. Her focus was on developing antennas which provide optimal performance in particular applications and in finding criteria to evaluate the performance of such antennas in the target applications. The work of Ms. Jalilvand thus represents an important contribution to the state of the art. I expect that her ideas and antennas will help researchers worldwide to come forward with their research on microwave based medical diagnostics. For Ms. Jalilvand, with her very good technical skills, I wish her success in her future career.
Prof. Dr.-Ing. Thomas Zwick - Institute Director

Application-Specific Broadband Antennas for Microwave Medical Imaging

Zur Erlangung des akademischen Grades eines

DOKTOR-INGENIEURS

von der Fakultät für
Elektrotechnik und Informationstechnik
des Karlsruher Instituts für Technologie (KIT)

genehmigte

DISSERTATION

von

M.Sc. Malyhe Jalilvand

geb. in Teheran, Iran

Tag der mündlichen Prüfung:	17.10.2016
Hauptreferent:	Prof. Dr.-Ing. Thomas Zwick
Korreferent:	Prof. Dr. rer. nat. Olaf Dössel

Contents

Abstract

This work presents research work about microwave medical imaging. Non-ionizing electromagnetic (EM) waves at microwave frequencies for medical diagnosis and imaging is emerging as a relatively low cost and low health risk alternative to the conventional imaging technologies.

Microwave technology is in general mature, portable and low cost, and therefore can offer the initial diagnosis of various life threatening conditions such as brain stroke while patients are still being on the way to a hospital in an ambulance. The required hardware of a microwave-based diagnosis system generally consists of a transmitter such as a vector network analyzer (VNA - portable available), an array of antennas (or sometimes a single antenna in sensing applications) and some switching network to switch between different antennas.

The success of a microwave imaging system depends, to a large extent, on technological aspects. In active near-field microwave medical imaging, transmitting and receiving antennas are placed in the close surrounding of the imaging object. Antenna array design in particular is known to have a direct impact on the image quality in both quantitative and qualitative imaging methods.

The choice of the antenna structure is very much dependent on the operating frequency range that itself is strongly dependent on the dielectric properties of the interface medium and the target application involved in the imaging scenario. Moreover, the exploited imaging technology usually demands special characteristics of the antennas. Therefore, antennas directly affect the accuracy of microwave imaging in both quantitative and qualitative approaches.

The goal of this work is the introduction of efficient antenna structures on the basis of the requirement of different microwave imaging methods; i.e. quantitative and qualitative microwave imaging techniques. To achieve this goal, several criteria are proposed for the evaluation of single element antenna structures for application in microwave tomography systems. The validity of the proposed criteria is further examined via simulated imaging results. Moreover, for qualitative Radar approaches, compact broadband antennas are proposed and evaluated for two target applications of breast cancer detection and stroke detection. the performance of the proposed antennas are evaluated in measurement scenarios.

Acronyms and Symbols

Acronyms

CF	coherence factor
Co-pol	co-polarization
CSF	cerebro-spinal fluid
CST	computer simulation technology
CT-scan	computed tomography scan
DAS	delay and sum
dB	decibel
E-Field	electric field
EM	electromagnetic
FCC	federal communications commission
FDTD	finite difference time domain
FE	finite element
FFT	fast Fourier transform
GHz	gigahertz
GPR	ground penetrating Radar
H-Field	magnetic field
IFFT	inverse fast Fourier transform
IO	imaging object

MATLAB	MATrix LABoratory
MHz	megahertz
MOM	method of moments
MRI	magnetic resonance imaging
MT	microwave tomography
PEG	Polyethylene Glycol
PET	positron emission tomography
RADAR	radio detection and ranging
RF	radio frequency
RMSE	root mean square error
SAR	specific absorption rate
SNR	signal to noise ratio
SCR	signal to clutter ratio
TM	transverse magnetic
TWI	through wall imaging
UWB	ultra-wide band
VNA	vector network analyser
X-pol	cross-polarization

Symbols and Constants

c_0	speed of light in vacuum ($\approx 2,997925 \cdot 10^8 m/s$)
d	distance
f	frequency
f_s	sampling frequency
k	wave number
n	sample
r_0	distance to a reference point in spherical coordinate
i	signal number in beamformer
x,y,z	Cartesian coordinate

Capital letters

B	magnetic flux density
D	dielectric flux density
E	electric field intensity
H	magnetic field intensity
J	conduction current density
M	number of signals in beamforming
N	number of samples
S11	input reflection coefficient at port 1
S21	forward transmission coefficient from port 1 to port 2
W_i	windowing coefficient in beamforming
X[n]	sampled input signal
$X_d[n]$	delayed input signal
Z[n]	sampled output signal

Greek symbols and Mathematical notation

α	attenuation constant
β	phase constant
ε	permittivity
ε_r	relative permittivity
ε_0	permittivity of free space ($8{,}854 \cdot 10^{-}12F/m$)
ε_∞	permittivity at the highest frequency in the Debye equation
ε_s	permittivity at the lowest frequency in the Debye equation
γ	complex propagation constant
Γ	reflection coefficient
T	transmission coefficient
λ	wavelength
λ_m	wavelength in a medium

μ	permeability
μ_0	permeability of free space $(4\pi \cdot 10^-7V.s/(A.m))$
π	Pi (3,14159...)
ρ	charge density
ρ_m	mass density
σ	conductivity
τ	time delay of signal
$\tau^{'}$	relaxation time in the Cole-Cole equation
ω	angular frequency
η_0	wave impedance in vacuum
η_m	wave impedance in a medium
j	imaginary unit j=$\sqrt{-1}$
∇	nabla
$\nabla.\vec{s}$	divergence of vector field
$\nabla \times \vec{s}$	rotation of vector field
$\|.\|$	absolute value
log	logarithm
A^T	transverse of matrix A

1 Introduction

This work presents research work about microwave medical imaging. Medical imaging in general has been long used for visualizing the interior of human body and is regarded as one very important tool for the diagnosis and identification of abnormalities in a noninvasive procedure. It has been widely used in many applications such as diagnosis of cancer and indeed during all the phases of cancer management, to name a few applications. In this chapter, first a short review of the conventional imaging modalities will be presented and the motivation behind the research on microwave imaging as an alternative or complementary approach for medical applications will be discussed. Furthermore, the state of the art of microwave medical imaging will be reviewed and the structure and goal of the work will be introduced.
Medical imaging facilities currently in service in today's hospital centers, mainly rely on ultrasound, X-rays and magnetic resonance imaging (MRI), computed tomography scan (CT scan) and positron emission tomography (PET). Some of these methods rely on ionizing radiation and provide clinical images with a variety of resolutions, implementation costs, and complexities ([8], [15]).
For instance, as discussed in [8] although MRI provides good resolution it is an expensive procedure. Another problem associated with MRI are measurement artifacts as a result of internal body movements such as heartbeat. CT scan uses X-ray radiation that is known to be ionizing and it fails at the imaging of the soft tissues. But generally it has a good spatial resolution. PET provides good information in case of soft tissues but it suffers from poor spatial resolution ([67]).

Moreover, the reported false-alarm rate of the aforementioned techniques for cancer detection is sometimes quite high. For example, X-ray mammography is normaly used for the detection of breast cancer where a high false negative rate (4-34%) and high false positive rate (70%) have been reported ([8] and [14]). Another main problem of the conventional imaging modalities is that they are not portable. Due to their bulky and expensive facilities, they are mainly available at large hospitals in big cities. A large population living far from urban areas have hardly access to these facilities at least in short time. This problem can lead to the death of the people in case of emergency situations such as head stroke.

Ultrasound is another conventional imaging technique that uses reflected sound waves to produce an image of the target under study. In case of human body imaging, it is most efficient for looking through organs and structures of soft tissues. Mineralized structures (e.g. bones) or air-filled organs (e.g. lungs) do not show up well on an ultrasound image ([74]). For instance for brain monitoring, ultrasound can only be best performed on babies before the bones of the skull have merged or on adults after the skull has been surgically opened.

Therefore, although the conventional techniques are widely used in medical field, there is room for alternative or supportive techniques to promise portable solutions and furthermore to help improve the diagnosis procedure regarding the safety issues, accuracy and reliability of the results.

1.1 Microwaves in medical applications

Non-ionizing electromagnetic (EM) waves at microwave frequencies for medical diagnosis and imaging is emerging as a relatively low cost and low health risk alternative to the conventional imaging technologies ([15], [49] and [8]). It is also sometimes considered a complementary technique for supporting and improving the available imaging modalities. Microwave imaging might enable frequent examinations of a women's breast enabling the detection of a possi-

ble cancer at the very early stage of development. The non-ionizing radiation of microwave signals in this case suggests a great advantage to the repeated conventional mammography.
Microwave technology is in general mature, portable and low cost, and therefore can offer the initial diagnosis of various life threatening conditions such as brain stroke while patients are still being on the way to a hospital in an ambulance. The required hardware of a microwave-based diagnosis system generally consists of a transmitter such as a vector network analyzer (VNA - portable available), an array of antennas (or sometimes a single antenna in sensing applications) and some switching network to switch between different antennas. This required hardware can be produced at a fraction of the price of other conventional diagnosis equipment and therefore it can facilitate the support of the patients in under-developing and developing countries.
Recently there has been a great progress in the development of efficient microwave imaging and sensing modalities (software and hardware) and lots of experimental prototypes have been suggested for different applications; e.g. breast tumor detection ([49] and [13]), pigs legs([68]), and canine heart ([69]). Furthermore, some pilot studies for clinical imaging prototypes have recently been published ([38] and [26]).
Another interesting approach in recent years has been that of hybrid imaging modalities [24], [80] and [66] to take advantage of the positive aspects of several imaging techniques. For instance, an interesting complementary imaging technique suggested for breast cancer detection is microwave-induced thermoacoustic imaging that combines the high contrast of microwave with the high resolution of ultrasound [80]. The hybrid techniques are beyond the scope of the work and will not be further discussed.
When talking about the application of microwaves in medical fields, we have to first distinguish between sensing and imaging applications. Although both approaches exploit non-ionizing EM waves at microwave frequencies for medical diagnosis, their ultimate goal is different.

1.1.1 Microwave sensing

In sensing applications, a microwave signal transmitted by an antenna is received either by the same antenna or a different antenna after scattering by an object. In such single-point applications, no image is constructed. The goal is to sense the change in amplitude or phase of the scattered signal and accordingly to comment on the status of the object. Instead they generate a graph between different sensed parameters. Some examples of the applications are detection of heartbeat, respiration and vital signs and recently an extensive research for the detection of stroke in human head ([50], [79] and [56]).
A review of some important research in microwave sensing can be found in [8]. The sensing applications are however beyond the scope of this work and will not be further discussed.

1.1.2 Microwave imaging

Imaging applications, on the other hand, result in a 2D or 3D image or map of the body. Depending on the imaging procedure, the images present either the location of a strong scatterer (relative energy map) or a map of the dielectric properties of the different tissues.
Microwave imaging itself can be divided into two major categories: passive and active techniques. For medical applications, only active techniques are significant since passive techniques do not allow full 3D imaging and have a far lower detection capability ([41]). As for 2D and 3D imaging, a variety of quantitative and qualitative imaging algorithms have been developed so far. This section provides a general overview of such methods and discusses the highlights of the positive and negative aspects of each category.

a. Quantitative imaging

   In quantitative imaging, also referred to as microwave tomography approach, the distribution of the dielectric properties (relative permittivity

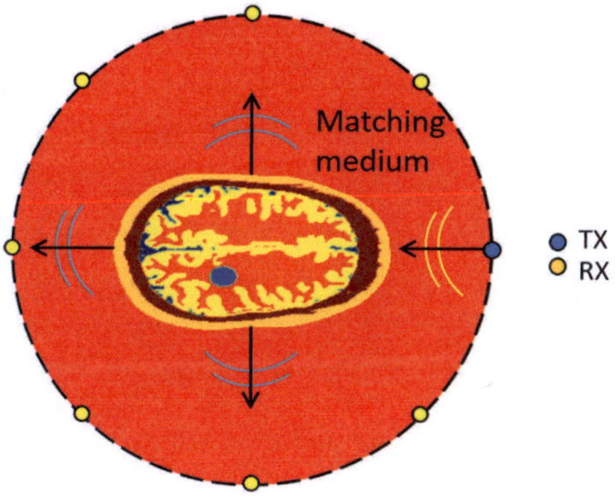

Fig. 1.1: The general microwave imaging setup; an imaging object (IO) immersed in a matching interface is surrounded by an array of antennas illuminating the IO with microwave signals and capturing the scattered fields around IO.

and conductivity) of various body tissues are reconstructed in the final image ([22], [40], [37] and [67]). The body to be imaged is usually surrounded by an array of antennas that illuminate the imaging object (IO) with microwave signals. For medical applications, usually the whole setup is immersed in a matching medium to reduce the reflection at the air-body interface and to couple the microwave signals efficiently to the IO. A principle drawing of a microwave imaging setup is shown in Fig. 1.1.

In medical applications, due to the large contrast of the dielectric properties of the different biological tissues, the inverse scattering problem is highly ill-posed. Therefore, linear approximations do not hold in practice and the inverse scattering problem has to be solved using nonlinear iterative algorithms. So far a variety of nonlinear iterative reconstruction algorithms have been proposed. The ultimate goal of all of them is the reconstruction of the dielectric properties of the imaging object ([8], [68] and [78]).

The reconstruction algorithms can be applied in frequency or time-domain using a broadband pulse [75]. They can further be applied at a single frequency or at multiple frequencies in a frequency hopping manner (e.g. in [58] and [5]). Frequency hopping can reduce the artifact level. However, due to the dispersive nature of the dielectric properties of the tissues, the frequency-dependence has to also be taken into account.

b. Qualitative imaging

In some medical imaging applications, it is not important to have the dielectric properties of the IO but instead the goal is merely to detect and localize a strong scatterer; e.g. a tumor in breast. For such applications there is no need to solve the computationally intensive inverse scattering problem (quantitative approach explained before). It will be discussed in the next chapter that a cancer has usually higher dielectric properties than normal tissues. In this case qualitative imaging algorithms can be applied to detect and localize the tumor. Various radar imaging algorithms have been so far developed to focus the tumor ([14], [4] and [71]). In all these techniques, to achieve a high resolution ultra-wideband (UWB) signals are exploited.

The implemented imaging setup resembles that of the quantitative imaging previously discussed (Fig. 1.1). Depending on the imaging procedure reflected signals (monostatic approach) or scattered signals in different directions (multistatic approach) are recorded. Imaging algorithms are used to focus the recorded signals. One major challenge of the qualitative approaches deals with the practical efficient procedure to focus the tumor response and get rid of the other not interesting responses such as the the skin response in case of breast cancer detection ([11]). Fig. 1.2 presents a general overview of the different microwave imaging techniques ([8]).

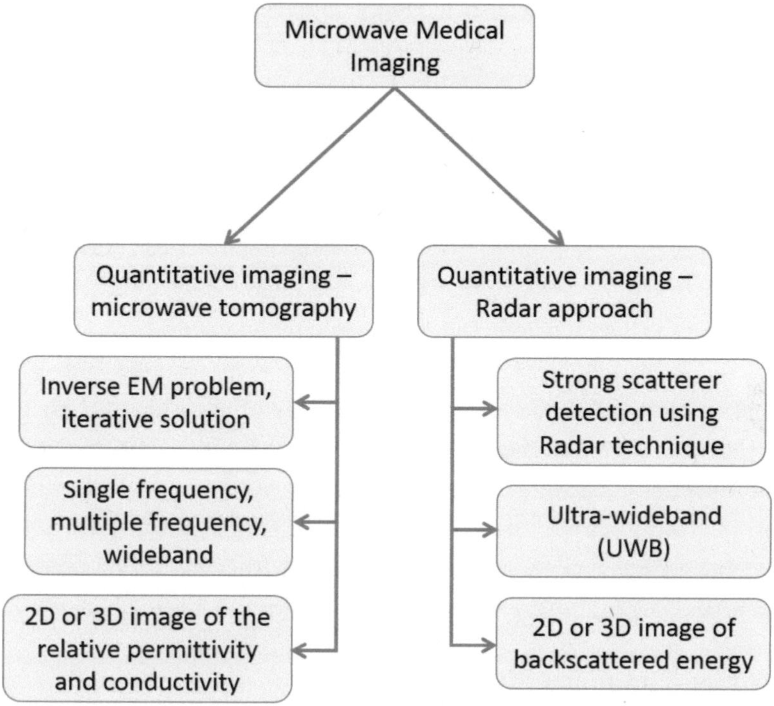

Fig. 1.2: Review of general microwave medical imaging methods.

1.2 Applications for microwave medical imaging

This section gives a short overview of some important applications of microwave medical imaging.

1.2.1 Breast imaging

Breast imaging is one of the most widely investigated applications of microwave medical imaging so far. The objective of this application is the detection and

localization of breast tumor that is known to have higher dielectric properties than the surrounding healthy tissues (10% to 400% higher- [30]).
The higher contrast of the tumor tissue makes it a significant scatterer and therefore as discussed before microwave Radar techniques (qualitative methods) can be in principle effectively applied. A lot of pioneer research has been reported for breast cancer detection via Radar-based techniques ([14], [4] and [71]). Moreover, due to the large contrast, the tumor can be relatively easily distinguished from the surrounding tissues using microwave tomography approaches [6] and [7]. Most of the investigations so far are based on numerical breast models and only very few investigations on actual women are so far reported [38].
The breast imaging setups use a planar, cylindrical or hemispherical antenna array implementation. The choice of the setup depends on the imaging approach; i.e. a cylindrical setup is used in microwave tomography methods whereas a hemispherical array is implemented in Radar-based imaging setups. It is been confirmed that a combination of an efficient hardware (antenna array) and a strong signal processing is absolutely critical for obtaining reliable imaging results.

1.2.2 Head imaging

The objective of human head imaging is the detection of damaged brain tissue due to ischemic or hemorrhagic stroke. The stroke results in either a blood clot (ischemic) or blood pool (hemorhagic) inside the brain. Due to the difference between the dielectric properties of normal brain tissues and stroke, the affected area can be detected using microwave imaging.
Some research has been reported in [61], [48], [65], [20] and [45] and [29] which concentrates on detecting a stroke in a simplified head model using microwave tomography imaging. In [65], a feasibility study on microwave stroke detection is performed using a realistic head model and numerical simulations. The effect of a stroke on the transmission coefficient is observed which is mainly on the received phase of the signal. Another feasibility assessment study on microwave

tomography for brain imaging is reported in [61]. A simple 2D head model is simulated at three frequencies and the dielectric profile of the model is reconstructed using nonlinear iterative tomography algorithms. In [48] the microwave Radar approach is used for stroke detection using broadband 2D antenna array positioned in air. According to the the research performed so far, it is believed that microwave technology has a potential for application in stroke detection.

1.2.3 Other microwave imaging applications

There are many other investigated applications using microwave technique such as imaging of bones [39], soft tissues and joints [64] and heart imaging [69]. The discussed topics in this work can in general be applied to all medical imaging applications.
[8] presents a general overview of current microwave medical imaging and sensing applications.

1.3 Antenna elements in microwave imaging systems

Microwaves are very sensitive and at the same time they undoubtedly carry invaluable information. The challenge is to efficiently retrieve this information. It is worth remembering, that for medical imaging applications, microwaves have to compete with already well-implemented imaging modalities.
The success of a microwave imaging system depends, to a large extent, on technological aspects. In active near-field microwave medical imaging, transmitting and receiving antennas are placed in the close surrounding of the imaging object. Antenna array design in particular is known to have a direct impact on the image quality in both quantitative and qualitative imaging methods [3] and [8].
The desired antenna structure has to efficiently direct microwave power towards the body for an optimum illumination and to have little sensitivity to the environmental interferences. Furthermore, the choice of the antenna structure is

very much dependent on the operating frequency range that itself is strongly dependent on the dielectric properties of the interface medium and the target application involved in the imaging scenario. Of great importance is the antenna dimension that limits the spatial sampling rate of the scattered field. Small-size antennas are especially interesting regarding the high sampling rate but difficult to match over a large bandwidth for achieving high spatial resolution in qualitative methods. In practical systems, bandwidth is usually sacrificed for the sake of size limitations. Especially the construction of an efficient antenna featuring high fractional bandwidth and small size is a great challenge at low frequencies [32] and [61].

Moreover, the exploited imaging technology usually demands special characteristics of the antennas. For instance, the accuracy of the quantitative methods, is directly influenced by the modeling including the antenna modeling in the forward problem setup; i.e. for tomographic imaging scenario, the image quality is ultimately related to how well the numerical model represents the actual measurement system. A Study in [70] shows that the number and location of antennas and the number of frequencies used in imaging procedure have a direct influence on the ill-posedness of the inverse problem in quantitative imaging methods.

Therefore, antennas directly affect the accuracy of microwave imaging in both quantitative and qualitative approaches. In the antenna design procedure, most of the time, a compromise must be found between contradictory aspects of antenna size, penetration depth and spatial resolution. As a result, depending on the considered application and the exploited imaging technology, there is a large degree of freedom to optimize a microwave medical imaging system.

1.4 Goal and outline of the work

In the light of the discussed challenges regarding the microwave imaging modalities for application in the medical field, the goal of this work is the introduction of efficient antenna structures on the basis of the requirement of different microwave imaging methods; i.e. quantitative and qualitative microwave imaging techniques.

To achieve this goal, several criteria are proposed for the evaluation of single element antenna structures for application in microwave tomography systems. The introduced criteria enable the evaluation and comparison of different antenna structures and further assist the development of efficient medical imaging systems using microwave technology. The validity of the proposed criteria is further examined via simulated imaging results. Moreover, for qualitative Radar approaches, compact broadband antennas are proposed for two target applications of breast cancer detection and stroke detection.

At this point it is necessary to emphasize that although the main focus of the research in this work is the application of microwave technology in medical field, the recommended solutions and especially the proposed criteria for the evaluation of antennas for different microwave imaging methods apply to other microwave imaging applications as well; namely through wall imaging (TWI), ground penetrating Radar (GPR) and industrial applications.

The organization of the work is as follows:

Chapter 2 covers a review of the concept of microwave medical imaging and explains the basis of the technique. It presents some basic dielectric properties of biological human body tissues (healthy and damaged tissues).

Chapter 3 deals with the considerations regarding the optimum microwave frequency range for medical imaging applications. Using an example scenario, it will be shown that the optimum frequency range is absolutely application-dependent. As a result, prior to any system deign and implementation, it is necessary to study the most important interaction of signals in microwave frequency range to the IO and to decide an optimum operational frequency. A 2D numerically realistic MRI derived head model is successfully imaged at a single frequency in the proposed spectrum using microwave tomography.

In Chapters 4 to 6 antenna structures are proposed and evaluated for quantitative and qualitative microwave imaging methods; namely full-wave 3D microwave tomography in Chapter 4, synthetic 3D microwave tomography in Chapter 5 and finally Radar beamforming in Chapter 6. For various imaging techniques the required specification of the antennas are first discussed and accordingly antenna structures are optimized for the specific application. At the end, optimal antenna structures are proposed for specified applications and imaging methods. Chapters 5 and 6 further include some evaluations of the proposed antennas for the target imaging applications.

The work will be wrapped up in Chapter 7 with a conclusion and discussion on the achievements of the research. This chapter will also include some suggestion for future extension of the current research. A list of the most important published achievements of this research can be found at the end of the dissertation (under own publication).

2 Fundamentals of microwave medical imaging

There is a need to investigate human anatomy and physiology for both healthy and abnormal cases. Medical imaging is an important tool to visualize the abnormalities in a mostly noninvasive procedure. Utilizing non-ionizing electromagnetic (EM) waves at microwave frequencies is regarded as an economical and low-risk imaging approach. The biological tissues of human body exhibit frequency-dependent (dispersive) characteristics at radio frequency (RF) spectrum. The RF signals interacting to our body will be generally attenuated and distorted passing through different layers. Therefore, when it comes to medical imaging using RF signals, it is of great importance to study and analyze the characteristics of tissues from the EM point of view.

In this chapter, the basic physical phenomena of EM wave propagation through a general lossy medium is discussed. Several important propagation characteristics such as the propagation constant, wave distortion, attenuation and penetration depth are generally reviewed in frequency range of DC to a few GHz. The human body is looked at from the EM point of view and the different biological layers are classified accordingly. After reviewing the EM properties of natural healthy tissues, the chapter will continue with the discussion of the changes of the EM properties of the normal tissues in case of abnormalities. The principle of microwave medical imaging will be discussed. Before further preceding to a deeper look at microwave medical imaging in the next chapters, some safety issues and concerns regarding the human body being exposed to microwave signals will be discussed.

2.1 Electromagnetic wave propagation through a general lossy medium

The propagation of electromagnetic wave are best described using maxwell's equations (as published by Maxwell in 1873) [57] and [2].

In case of a linear media (ε and μ independent of $\vec{E}$ and $\vec{H}$), the Maxwell equations in phasor form can be written as:

$$\nabla\times\vec{E}=-jw\mu\vec{H} \tag{2.1}$$

$$\nabla\times\vec{H}=jw\varepsilon\vec{E}+\vec{J} \tag{2.2}$$

$$\nabla\cdot\vec{D}=\rho \tag{2.3}$$

$$\nabla\cdot\vec{B}=0 \tag{2.4}$$

The constitutive relations are as follows:

$$\vec{D}=\varepsilon\vec{E} \tag{2.5}$$

$$\vec{B}=\mu\vec{H} \tag{2.6}$$

where ε and μ are the so called permittivity and permeability of the medium. They might be complex tensors depending on the medium through which the EM waves propagate.

In general, a homogeneous, isotropic and lossy medium can be thoroughly described using its complex permittivity and permeability that can be written as follows:

$$\varepsilon=\varepsilon_0(\varepsilon'-j\varepsilon'')=\varepsilon_0\varepsilon_r \tag{2.7}$$

$$\mu=\mu_0(\mu'-j\mu'')=\mu_0\mu_r \tag{2.8}$$

$\varepsilon_0 = 8.85 \times 10^{-12}$ and $\mu_0 = 4\pi \times 10^{-7}$ are the intristic permittivity and permeability of vacuum.
ε'' is responsible for the dielectric and conductive losses of the medium. In most of the human tissues the conductive currents are however dominant. ε_r is the so called relative permittivity of the medium (generally a complex value). Biological tissues are furthermore assumed to be non-magnetic and therefore throughout this work μ'' is considered to be zero.
For a medium conductivity σ, a corresponding conduction current density $\vec{J}$ exists that is proportional to the $\vec{E}$ vector according to:

$$\vec{J} = \sigma \vec{E} \tag{2.9}$$

Equation (2.2) can be re-written as:

$$\begin{aligned} \nabla \times \vec{H} &= jw\varepsilon \vec{E} + \vec{J} \\ &= jw\varepsilon_0\varepsilon_r \vec{E} + \sigma \vec{E} \\ &= jw\varepsilon_0[\varepsilon_r - j\frac{\sigma}{w\varepsilon_0}]E \end{aligned} \tag{2.10}$$

Therefore, the modified complex permittivity can be expressed as:

$$\varepsilon = \varepsilon_0(\varepsilon_r - j\frac{\sigma}{w\varepsilon_0}) \tag{2.11}$$

To define other important propagation parameters, we need to have the wave equation. For a source-free medium ($\vec{M} = 0$), the wave equation can be derived as follows starting from (2.1):

$$\begin{aligned} \nabla \times \vec{E} &= -jw\mu_0 \vec{H} \\ \nabla \times \nabla \times \vec{E} &= -jw\mu_0 \nabla \times \vec{H} \\ \nabla(\nabla . \vec{E}) - \nabla^2 \vec{E} &= w^2\mu_0\varepsilon_0[\varepsilon_r - j\frac{\sigma}{w\varepsilon_0}] \vec{E} \end{aligned} \tag{2.12}$$

that is:

$$\nabla^2 \vec{E} + w^2 \mu_0 \varepsilon_0 [\varepsilon_r - j\frac{\sigma}{w\varepsilon_0}] \vec{E} = 0 \tag{2.13}$$

To simplify the above equation, the wave number in a lossy medium is defined as:

$$k = w\sqrt{\mu_0 \varepsilon_0 [\varepsilon_r - j\frac{\sigma}{w\varepsilon_0}]} \tag{2.14}$$

Here, the complex wave propagation constant for the medium can be defined as:

$$\gamma = \alpha + j\beta = jk = jw\sqrt{\mu_0 \varepsilon_0 [\varepsilon_r - j\frac{\sigma}{w\varepsilon_0}]} \tag{2.15}$$

α and β are the attenuation and phase constants, respectively. By separating the real and imaginary parts of the right side of the above equation they can be more specifically derived as follows:

$$\alpha = \frac{w}{c_0}\sqrt{\frac{\varepsilon_r}{2}[\sqrt{1 + (\frac{\sigma}{w\varepsilon_0\varepsilon_r})^2} - 1]} \tag{2.16}$$

$$\beta = \frac{w}{c_0}\sqrt{\frac{\varepsilon_r}{2}[\sqrt{1 + (\frac{\sigma}{w\varepsilon_0\varepsilon_r})^2} + 1]} \tag{2.17}$$

2.1.1 Attenuation constant

It is obvious that the existence of conductive loss (σ) leads to a non-zero attenuation constant and correspondingly introduces losses to the propagation of the signals.

According to (2.13) and (2.15) the wave equation for an electric field with only $\widehat{x}$ component becomes:

$$\frac{\partial^2 E_x}{\partial^2 x} - \gamma^2 E_x = 0 \tag{2.18}$$

which has the solution:

$$E_x(z) = E^+ e^{-\gamma z} + E^- e^{\gamma z} \tag{2.19}$$

The propagation factor of the positive travelling wave is of the form:

$$e^{-\gamma z} = e^{-\alpha z} e^{-\beta z} \tag{2.20}$$

It represents an exponentially damping wave travelling in +z direction with a phase velocity of $v_p = \frac{w}{\beta}$ and a wavelength of $\lambda = \frac{2\pi}{\beta}$. α, the attenuation constant, determines the rate of the decay of the wave. Assuming a distance of 1 meter it can be expressed in dB as follows:

$$D_{(dB/m)} = 20.log_{10}(e^{-\alpha}) = -20.\alpha.log_{10}(e) = 8.686.\alpha \tag{2.21}$$

2.1.2 Penetration depth

Another very important parameter is the penetration depth or the so called skin depth. As the name implies, it refers to the penetration capability of the EM wave into a general lossy medium. It is defined as the depth at which the strength of the field (magnitude) decays to $\frac{1}{e}$ of the field value at the surface of the medium; that is:

$$\delta_p = \frac{1}{\alpha} = \frac{c_0}{w\sqrt{\frac{\varepsilon_r}{2}[\sqrt{1+(\frac{\sigma}{w\varepsilon_0\varepsilon_r})^2} - 1]}} \tag{2.22}$$

2.1.3 Wave impedance

The wave impedance in a lossy medium can be estimated from:

$$\eta_m = \sqrt{\frac{\mu}{\varepsilon}} = \sqrt{\frac{\mu_0}{\varepsilon_0[\varepsilon_r - j\frac{\sigma}{w\varepsilon_0}]}} = \frac{\eta_0}{\sqrt{[\varepsilon_r - j\frac{\sigma}{w\varepsilon_0}]}} \tag{2.23}$$

η_0 is the intrinsic wave impedance of vacuum and is equal to 120π. Since the permittivity and conductivity are frequency-dependent ($\varepsilon_r(w)$ and $\sigma(w)$), it turns out that the wave impedance also varies with frequency.
From the discussion above and following the introduction of the most important wave propagation parameters, it turns out that with the knowledge of the complex relative permittivity of a medium (dielectric properties of a medium), in principle it is possible to estimate the phase constant, attenuation, penetration depth and wave impedance. Therefore the dielectric properties of human biological tissues are the basis of the analysis of wave propagation and its interaction with the human body. In the next section, we'll have a look at the dielectric properties of the biological human body tissues.

2.2 Dielectric properties of biological tissues

The dielectric properties of biological tissues are the key to analyzing and understanding the different possible interactions of EM waves and the human body. Therefore a good knowledge about the dielectric properties of biological tissues is of great importance.
An early review of the dielectric properties of human tissues is presented in [16]. The measurements of the dielectric properties of the tissues range from in-vivo to ex-vivo techniques as presented by Gabriel in [16]. Different types of tissues, including both healthy and abnormal tissues, have distinct dielectric properties (relative permittivity and conductivity). These differences originate from the different water-content of the various tissues which results in a variation of the scattered signals by the tissues. Even the dielectric properties of a single biological tissue are frequency dependent. Therefore, not only various tissues exhibit different dielectric properties, these properties of a single tissue vary also versus frequency.
To model the frequency dispersive nature of a biological tissue, one can use the Debye model or the Cole-Cole model. Using either of these two estimation mo-

dels, the dielectric properties of human tissues based on experimental databases can be estimated and predicted.

2.2.1 Debye model

According to [16], one possible model to predict the frequency-dependent dielectric properties of biological tissues is the Debye model. It is a rather straightforward first-oder approximation that predicts the complex relative permittivity of a single tissue as a function of frequency. The equation is as follows:

$$\varepsilon = \varepsilon_0(\varepsilon_r - j\frac{\sigma}{w\varepsilon_0}) = \varepsilon_\infty + \frac{\varepsilon_s - \varepsilon_\infty}{1 + jw\tau'} \tag{2.24}$$

ε_∞ is the saturated permittivity at very high frequencies, ε_s is the static permittivity at very low frequencies. $\Delta\varepsilon = \varepsilon_s - \varepsilon_\infty$ is described as the magnitude of the dispersion and finally τ' is a relaxation time constant.

The Debye model is a first order approximation and gives only a rough estimate of the dielectric properties of the tissues. The model proves to fail at correctly predicting the dielectric properties in broadband frequency ranges.

2.2.2 Cole - Cole model

The spectrum of the tissues can be more accurately described by the higher-order approximation model from Cole-Cole [16]. The Cole-Cole dispersion model is as follows:

$$\varepsilon(w) = \varepsilon_\infty + \sum_n \frac{\Delta\varepsilon_n}{1 + (jw\tau_n)^{(1-\alpha_n)}} + \frac{\sigma_i}{jw\varepsilon_0} \tag{2.25}$$

α_n is the distribution parameter and is a measure of the frequency dispersion. σ_i is an added conductivity term ([16]).

With a choice of appropriate parameters corresponding to each tissue, 2.25 can be applied to predict the frequency-dependent dielectric characteristic of a single tissue over a desired range of frequencies. Fig. 2.1 shows the relative permittivity

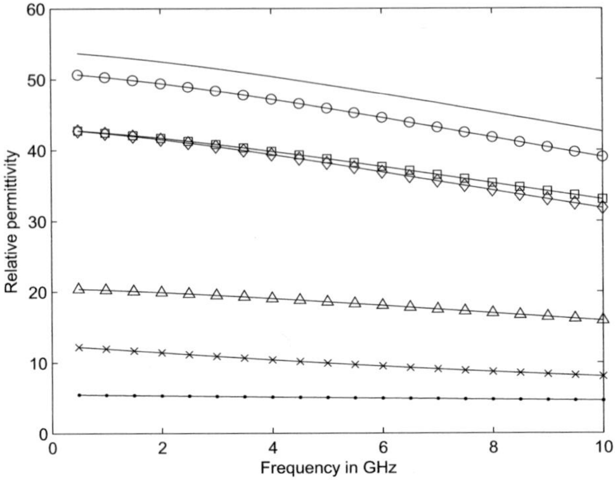

(a)

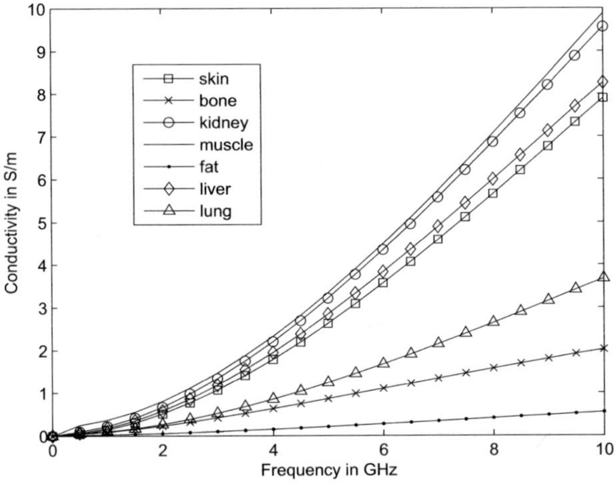

(b)

Fig. 2.1: The relative permittivity and conductivity of some biological tissues as predicted by the Cole-Cole approximation over a broad range of frequencies.

and conductivity of a couple of biological tissues at a broad frequency range as predicted by the Cole-Cole formula.

2.3 Examples of abnormalities of human tissues

When an abnormality occurs in a tissue, the dielectric properties of that tissue change. This alternation of relative permittivity and conductivity can be indeed sensed using microwaves. This is the basic of microwave medical imaging.
Apart from the different water content of healthy and abnormal tissues, a variety of other factors exist that are proven to be responsible for the difference in the dielectric properties of healthy tissues and abnormalities eg. inflammation causing the breakdown of the cell membrane. In the following, we look deeply at two major life-threatening abnormalities affecting many people in the world: breast cancer and head stroke.

2.3.1 Breast cancer

Breast cancer is one of the most common cancer in the world. More and more women are anticipated to be diagnosed with breast cancer in future. Studies performed since the 1960s, show that regular screening for the early diagnosis of the breast cancer can reduce the growth rate of the disease. Current clinical screening techniques suffer from limitations for breast cancer detection ([49] and [8]). These limitations motivated the researches all over the world to investigate alternative or supportive approaches for breast screening. In particular, techniques relying on EM detection have been recently receiving special interest. The detection of breast cancer using microwave technology relies on the contrast between the dielectric properties of normal breast and tumor tissues.
Lazebnik ([30]) performed a large scale study on the ex-vivo measured dielectric properties of normal and malignant tissues over the frequency range from 0.5 to 20 GHz. According to this study, normal breast tissues are divided into three groups: 1) low (0-30%); 2) average (31-84%); 3) high (85-100%) adipose (fat)

tissue content. The results of the study enable the representation of the dispersive dielectric properties of each tissue type using Cole-Cole model 2.25.

Fig. 2.2 shows the dielectric properties of the three normal breast tissue types together with the dielectric properties of a ex-vivo measured malignant tissue. It is concluded that the dielectric properties of normal breast tissue vary significantly over frequency and moreover, they heavily depend on the adipose level. The contrast in dielectric properties between an adipose-dominant tissue and a tumor follows a ratio of 10:1. This contrast, however, falls down to approximately 10% between a low adipose tissue and malignant tissue. The contrast between a normal breast tissue and tumor is however in all cases sufficiently large to be sensed by microwave imaging.

2.3.2 Head stroke

Stroke or brain attack remains an important and time-sensitive health concern in the world. It refers to a disturbance in the blood flow leading to malfunctions of the brain. The injury is regarded as a high risk concern having the potential to be fatal (accounted for 1 in every 16 deaths in the USA and second major cause of human death in the whole world) or sometimes leading to lifelong disabilities [60], [23] and [47].

Acute ischemic stroke is known to be the major type of stroke. It is the consequence of a blockage caused by a local clot in the blood circulation route interrupting the blood supply to some part of the brain. If not treated in time this reduction of blood supply may lead to irreversible damage of the brain tissues. Another category of brain malfunction as a result of blood flow disturbance is that of hemorrhagic stroke. This would be the consequence of bleeding somewhere inside the brain which may be due to a rupture of a vessel.

The symptoms of stroke are varied and range from weakness, dizziness, slurred speech, problems with reading, etc. A suspected stroke is an emergency situation and regarding the fact that the two mentioned kinds of strokes share similar

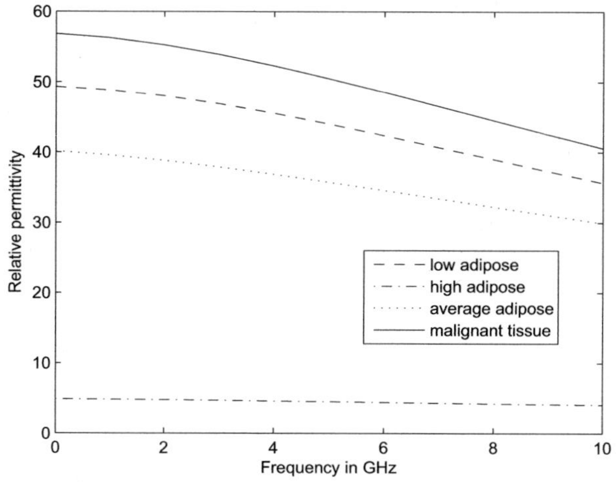

(a)

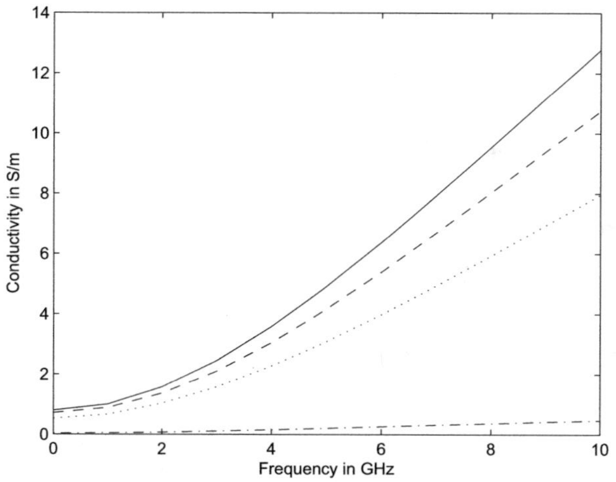

(b)

Fig. 2.2: The relative permittivity and conductivity of three categories of normal breast tissue and malignant tissues over a broad range of frequencies.

symptoms however require totally different measures, fast and reliable diagnosis techniques within the early hours since the first symptoms show up, are vital for a successful treatment.

Typical stroke diagnosis is carried out using a neurological examination followed by medical imaging techniques the most common ones for this application are computed tomography (CT scan) and magnetic resonance imaging (MRI) [47]. Although these current imaging techniques are efficient in terms of identification of the type and location of stroke, they suffer from not being fast, cost effective and portable and so are limited to major hospitals and are not available in all medical clinics. This very negative fact invokes the main motivation of looking for alternative imaging techniques speeding up the procedure in terms of availability of portable diagnosis devices in ambulances and small clinics to initiate the necessary treatment procedure with less delay.

One efficient portable imaging instrumentation nowadays is ultrasound. For this specific application of stroke detection, the major insurmountable obstacle for ultrasound systems is that the skull bone has a high acoustic impedance leading to nearly 100% reflection at the boundary so that nearly no intensity is transmitted into the brain. Skull has also a high sound propagation speed compared to soft tissues, and has a variable thickness that distorts the wave propagation and destroys the focus of a beam. For imaging of the human head in general ultrasound is not a viable technology [74].

Biological tissues of human body can be categorized into two major groups regarding the water content. The high water content tissues such as skin, muscle, brain and low water content tissues like fat and bones. Human head consisting of skin, skull and brain lies in the high-contrast medium category which is a difficult environment to be imaged using microwave techniques (Fig. 2.3). Therefore for a successful detection of stroke, a highly efficient imaging system integrating high performance antennas, detectors and sensors together with novel image reconstruction and classification algorithms are necessary to cope with the high attenuation and scattering of the signals propagating in brain tissues. This subject will be discussed more in the next chapters.

2.4 Safety concerns of exposure to microwave energy

Thermal effects are the proven dangers of exposure to electromagnetic radiation. Human body absorbs radio frequency (RF) and microwave radiation and turns it to heat. The heating occurs inside the body and can not be felt from outside (as in the case of microwave oven). Most dangerous human organs are brain, eyes and the stomach. Therefore, when it comes to using EM waves for medical applications, it is of great importance to determine reliable safety levels in order to prevent exposure to harmful power levels [57].
Specific absorption rate (SAR) ist one exposure limit set by the Federal Communications Commission (FCC) which measures the amount of the dissipated power (heat) in a unit of tissue mass. SAR is defined as:

$$SAR = \frac{\sigma}{2\rho_m} \left|\vec{E}\right|^2 W/kg \tag{2.26}$$

where σ is the conductivity of the tissue (S/m), ρ_m is the tissue density (kg/m^3) and $\vec{E}$ is the electric field inside the tissue. The assigned SAR limit by FCC in the frequency range of 100 KHz to 10 GHz is $1.6W/kg$ averaged over 1g of tissue. In Europa, however, the limits are set at $2W/kg$ averaged over 10g of tissue.

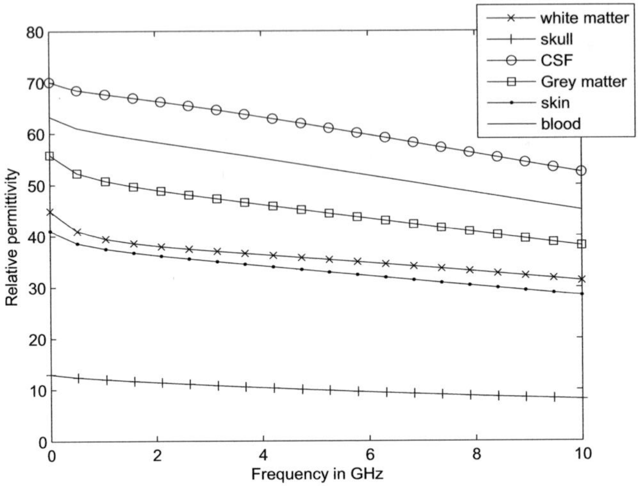

(a)

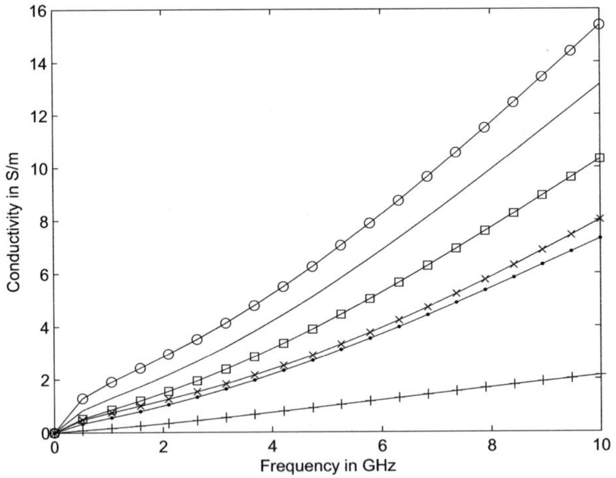

(b)

Fig. 2.3: The relative permittivity and conductivity of human head tissues versus frequency; Cole-cole model.

3 Specifications and requirements for microwave medical imaging

In this chapter, some active microwave imaging modalities are reviewed. It will be discussed that the specification of a microwave imaging system depends on one side on the target imaging application and on the other side on the employed imaging method (i.e. quantitative or qualitative approach).
For an example scenario of head imaging using microwaves, the most important interactions of the signals to a multilayer human head model are studied. The ultimate goal is to comment on the frequency requirement of a microwave imaging system for the detection of stroke in human head. The possibility of detecting a hemorrhagic stroke using the microwave quantitative method is further examined using a numerically realistic head model (MRI-derived model).

3.1 Microwave imaging methods

3.1.1 On the importance of a matching interface

In microwave medical imaging, the complete imaging setup is usually immersed in an interface medium with complex permittivity of ε_m called a matching medium. The idea behind using a matching medium is to efficiently couple the EM energy to the body and minimize the reflections at the air-body interface. Furthermore, since the resolution of a microwave imaging system is wavelength-dependent, by applying a matching medium the imaging resolution is increased according to:

$$\lambda_m = \frac{\lambda_0}{\sqrt{\varepsilon_m}} \tag{3.1}$$

where λ_0 is the wavelength of the microwave signal in air.
A lossy matching medium will also limit the reflections off the tank boundaries. Losses further ensure that the signals collected by receivers are mainly dominated by the scattering of the imaging object and that all the other multi-paths are negligible.
On the other hand, a lossy matching liquid attenuates both the unwanted reflections and the main target signal, simultaneously. As a result, a high dynamic range and signal-to-noise ratio is essential to capture the target reflections above the noise level. However, considering the higher permittivity of biological tissues compared to air, the matching medium is considered as an optimal way of coupling most of the microwave energy into an IO and avoiding the high losses at the air-body interface.
For 2D and 3D microwave imaging, both quantitative and qualitative imaging algorithms have been developed. In the following we will have a look at some such imaging methods.

3.1.2 Quantitative microwave tomography

Microwave tomography (MT) is an imaging modality that has a broad range of applications e.g. industrial non-destructive testing, through-wall imaging, landmine detection, detection of defects and cracks in construction materials and biomedical imaging. Ever since the introduction of the technique in the late 70âs, there has been a non-stop effort in the development of sophisticated algorithms and practical measurement systems in the frequency range from a few hundred Megahertz up to a few Gigahertz [22].
In this imaging approach, the body to be imaged is surrounded by an array of transmit and receive antennas. The body is then in turn illuminated by the mi-

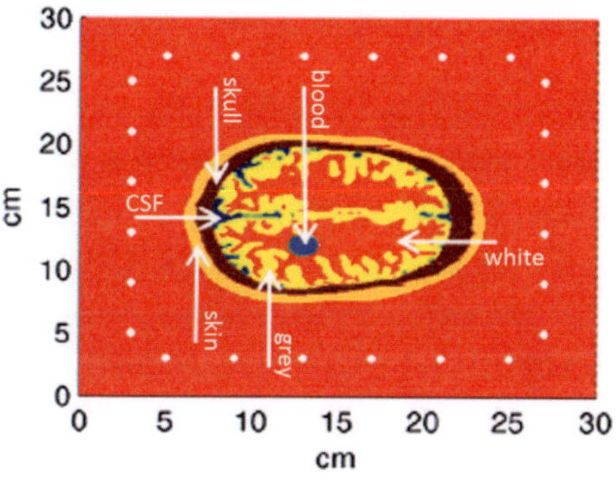

Fig. 3.1: Imaging setup in microwave tomography method; an IO with unknown relative permittivity and conductivity is surrounded by an array of antennas.

crowave signal of a transmit antenna and the scattered signals at different observation points are recorded by all the receive antennas (Fig. 3.1).

The ultimate goal of a MT imaging system for biomedical applications is the quantitative reconstruction (2D or 3D) of the complex dielectric properties of the IO (relative permittivity and conductivity). In the medical field, a lot of progress has been reported on the detection of breast cancer yet many other applications have also emerged e.g. stroke detection and bone imaging [7], [46] and [39].

The general image reconstruction procedure in microwave tomography is summarized in the block diagram of Fig. 3.2. Microwave tomography imaging of biomedical bodies includes the following steps:

1. The final goal of MT imaging is the reconstruction of the relative permittivity and conductivity of the biological object. As can be seen in Fig. 3.1, an IO is surrounded by an array of antennas. With the antennas acting sequentially as transmitters and receivers, a number of measured scattered signals are recorded at several observation points. The goal is to figure out a unique solution for the inversion problem of determining the relative

permittivity and conductivity of the object using the measured scattered signals.

2. After performing the measurement and obtaining the measured scattered signals from the object, the measurement setup is simulated in a numerical solver which is referred to as forward solver. Different numerical analysis techniques can be used as forward solver. Examples are the method of moments (MOM), finite element (FE), finite difference time domain (FDTD) [63]. A numerical model of the measurement setup is generated in the forward solver and the simulation domain is divided into mesh cells.

3. The first step in the reconstruction procedure, is the assignment of an initial relative permittivity and conductivity to the different mesh cells of the simulation model in the forward solver (initial guess). Usually, the whole mesh cells are initially assigned the same dielectric properties as the surrounding matching medium.

4. With the assigned initial guess, the numerical simulation in the forwards solver runs and scattered signals are simulated (first iteration).

5. The measurement signals are correspondingly compared to the obtained simulated scattered signals and the error is estimated.

6. In this step, the relative permittivity and conductivity of the different mesh cells in the simulation model of forward solver are updated to minimize the error between the measured and simulated scattered signals. For medical imaging, nonlinear iterative optimization algorithms are applied. One example of the optimization techniques is the nonlinear iterative Gauss-Newton approach [22].

7. After applying an optimization technique, the dielectric properties of all the mesh cells in the numerical model are updated. Afterwards, with the

new estimated dielectric properties, the forward solver is re-simulated and another set of simulated scattered signals are estimated.

8. The procedure is repeated iteratively until the error converges (at this point updating the dielectric properties of the mesh cells, doesn't improve the results anymore).

The above discussed image reconstruction procedure can be applied either at a single frequency or over a wideband spectrum (the so called frequency hopping technique [58]). In a frequency hopping approach, ignoring the frequency dispersion of the different tissues, the results obtained at one frequency are used as a starting guess for an upper frequency. This way it is possible to decrease the artifact level especially in the reconstructed conductivity profile of the body.

3.1.3 Qualitative Radar imaging

In some medical imaging applications, such as breast cancer detection, the aim is not to obtain a map of the dielectric properties of the object but only to determine if there is a tumor inside the body or not and to localize it. In such cases, no computationally intensive iterative reconstruction algorithms are necessary. As discussed in the previous chapter, breast tumor has usually higher dielectric properties than the healthy surrounding tissues that makes it a strong scatterer. Various Radar imaging algorithms can be utilized to focus the tumor ([51], [4] and [14]). These techniques are similar to quantitative approaches in that the object is again surrounded by an array of antennas. Each antenna transmits an Ultra Wideband (UWB) signal (short pulse at a time) to guarantee a good spatial resolution.

In Radar imaging, the backscattered signals contain not only the tumor response, they also include the artifact of skin response and the response from all other tissues we are not interested in (interference signal). Therefore, some preprocessing needs to be performed to extract the pure tumor response from the recorded signal. For this purpose several pre-processing algorithms are proposed in the literature [11] and [27].

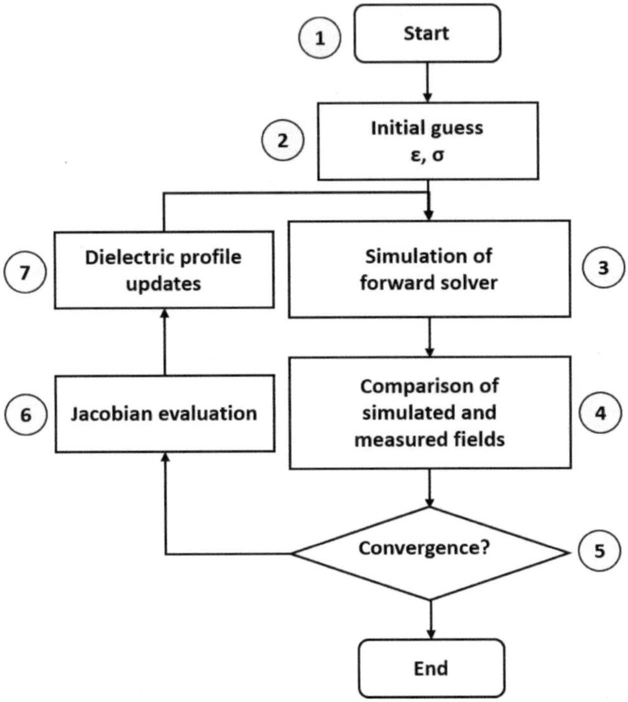

Fig. 3.2: The flowchart of a general image reconstruction algorithm in microwave tomography.

After the removal of unwanted skin-response, the imaging procedure includes the following steps:

1. The pre-processed backscattered signal at each antenna is integrated over time (if the measurements are performed in the frequency domain, they have to be converted into the time domain using inverse fast Fourier transform (IFFT)).

2. All the integrated waveforms are then time-shifted to focus a single specific pixel in the imaging domain. By adjusting appropriate time-shifts the beamformer is scanned to different focal points inside the IO.

3. The time-shifted signals from all the antennas are afterwards coherently summed to obtain the associated intensity of each synthetic focal point in the imaged body.

4. The energy of the resultant signal is a single value showing the backscattered signal energy at different locations inside the IO.

3.2 Specification of microwave medical imaging - example application of stroke detection

When it comes to the required specification of a microwave medical imaging setup, the target application needs to be first specified. This is because the specification (such as frequency range, antenna type, dynamic range, etc) is application-dependent. Therefore, at the beginning of designing a system for medical imaging, the target application needs to be deeply studied and only after that we can comment on the hardware and software requirement of the ultimate imaging system.
Above all, the operating frequency range is very determining as it directly influences both the hardware and software of the imaging system. To decide the optimum frequency range for a specific application, the interaction of microwave signals to the target IO needs to be previously studied. As a general rule, in microwave imaging a lower frequency of the spectrum allows good penetration into the IO however due to the large wavelength at these frequencies they yield a poor resolution. A higher spectrum, on the other hand, generally results in a good resolution but it fails at penetrating deep inside the IO. Therefore, to decide the optimum frequency range of a Radar for a specific application the interaction of microwave signals to the target IO needs to be studied first.

In the following, as an example application, the required bandwidth of a microwave imaging system for the detection of stroke in a human head is studied. The procedure includes looking at a human head from electromagnetic points of view, i.e the dielectric properties of brain, and the interaction of broadband microwave signals to the different layers of a human head. Specially the attenuation of individual head tissues, the effective penetration depth of the microwave signals inside the head model at different frequencies, the transmission and reflection of the signals at the interface between adjacent layers will be estimated. At the end of the analysis, an optimum frequency range is proposed for human head imaging.

3.2.1 Microwaves for head imaging

A human head consists mainly of five layers including skin, skull, cerebro-spinal fluid (CSF), gray matter and white matter. The layers are generally dispersive and vary vastly regarding the water-content, i.e a human head includes the very low water-content skull as well as the high water-content CSF and brain [16]. Microwave imaging exploits the difference between the dielectric properties of the tissues to detect and localize any malfunctions inside the brain. Therefore, an efficient penetration of microwave signals into the human head in order to distinguish the different layers is an extreme challenge.

Tabelle 3.1: Typical thickness of human head different tissues

Tissue	Thickness (mm)
Skin	5
Skull	7
CSF	5
Gray matter	22
White matter	30

For the analysis of the interactions between microwave signals and the human head, a planar multilayer structure is analytically studied. The model consists of six planar layers infinite in size whose arrangement is shown in Fig. 3.3. The dispersive dielectric properties of the layers are obtained from the Cole-Cole formula previously mentioned in Chapter 2. Each layer is assigned its typical thickness similar to the real biological one as mentioned in the literature (Table 3.1); [61]. A hemorrhagic stroke approximated as a blood layer is inserted deep inside the multilayer head model inside the white matter (Fig. 3.3).

To begin the analysis, we look at some individual properties of the layers. Fig. 3.4 (a) presents the attenuation constant of each tissue as a function of frequency up to 10 GHz. As can be seen in the figure, a broadband signal will be attenuated differently inside different tissues. Furthermore, the amount of attenuation a broadband signal experiences depends very much on the frequency since the tissues are very dispersive. For instance, inside the gray matter tissue, the attenuation of 4 dB/cm at 2 GHz increases to 6 dB/cm at 4 GHz. Therefore, considering a broadband signal, the different attenuation at different frequencies will lead to the distortion of the signal.

Another characteristic of the individual head tissues is the penetration depth. Fig. 3.4 (b) displays the estimated penetration depth inside the different head tissues versus frequency. It is observed in the figure, that as the frequency increases the signal can hardly penetrate inside the tissues. At frequencies above 4 GHz the penetration inside the brain decreases to only a few cm.

On the other hand, in microwave imaging the resolution is determined by the wavelength. Although generally speaking higher frequencies are specially interesting to achieve high resolution in medical imaging, the utilization of higher frequencies is limited due to the large attenuation of the tissues at higher frequencies and the lower penetration capability of the microwave signals inside the tissues as the frequency increases.

In conclusion, for a successful imaging using microwave signals, some compromise needs to be done to enable efficient imaging i.e. enough penetration and good resolution. For the example of the detection of stroke utilizing microwave imaging, the interaction of microwave signals as they penetrate into different head layers are discussed in the following parts of this chapter. The goal is to estimate the transfer function of the multilayer head model at different frequencies. Considering the practical concerns and limitations, only after this analysis we would be able to recommend an efficient bandwidth for head imaging using microwaves.

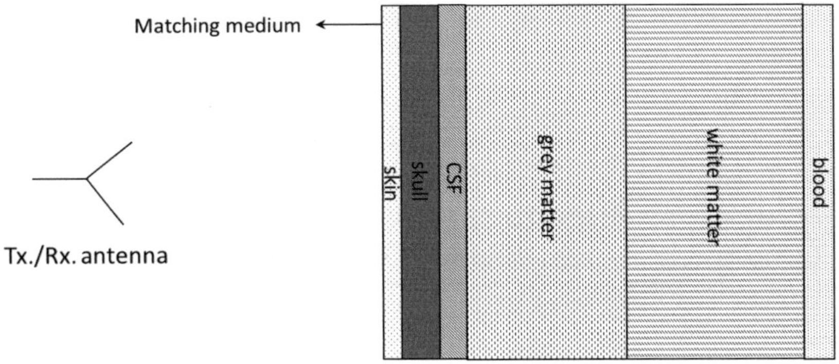

Fig. 3.3: The planar multilayer head model for ray tracing analysis.

3.2.2 Interaction of microwave signals to a multilayer head model

When a microwave signal impinges an interface, the waves will be generally diffracted. Diffraction is a complex physical phenomena and to analyze it exactly, complicated numerical codes are necessary. Diffraction refers to EM signals being scattered, partially transmitted at an interface and partially reflected. To study the interaction of microwave signals to the planar multilayer head model of Fig. 3.3, the following three first-order scattering phenomena are taken into account [57]:

1. attenuation of the signals as they propagate through the layers,

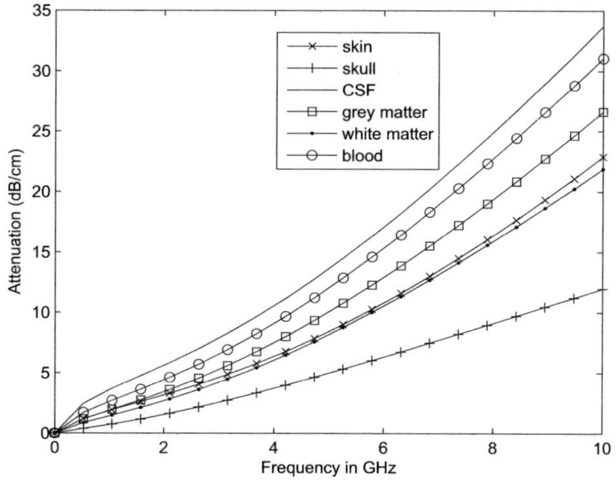

(a)

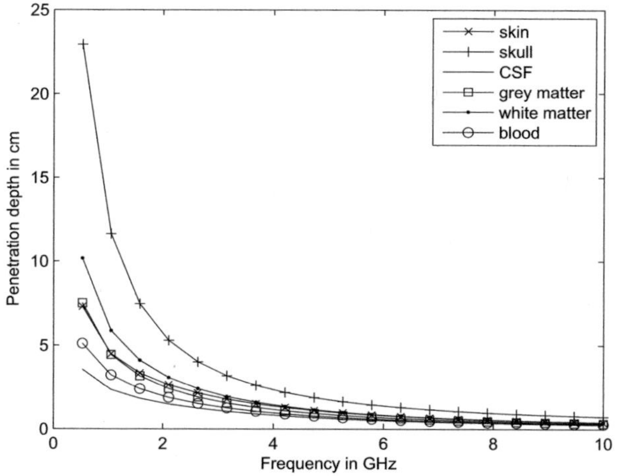

(b)

Fig. 3.4: (a) The attenuation constant of human head tissues over frequency. (b) The penetration depth inside human head tissues over frequency.

2. partial transmission of the signals at the interface from one layer to the adjacent layer,

3. partial reflection of the signals at an interface back towards the transmitter,

To estimate the transmission and reflection coefficients at an interface between two mediums of relative complex permittivity of ε_{r1} and ε_{r2} the following formulation valid for normal incidence can be used [57]:

$$\Gamma_1 = \frac{\eta_2 - \eta_1}{\eta_2 + \eta_1} \tag{3.2}$$

$$T_{21} = \frac{2\eta_2}{\eta_2 + \eta_1} \tag{3.3}$$

$$\eta_i = \frac{\eta_0}{\sqrt{\varepsilon_{ri}}} \tag{3.4}$$

η_0 is the intrinsic wave impedance of vacuum. Knowing the corresponding transmission and reflection coefficients of all the layers, it is possible to estimate the amount of transmitted and reflected energy at each interface (Fig. 3.5). Inside each layer, the waves undergo attenuation that can be estimated using the specific attenuation constant of the different tissues (Fig. 3.4 (a)). The penetration depth inside each tissue is further estimated and displayed in (Fig. 3.4 (b)). This, enables us to perform a simple analysis to predict the interaction of the microwave signals to the simplified multilayer head model of Fig. 3.3 approximately. An ideal point-source antenna radiating a 0 dBm plane wave in the frequency range of DC to 5 GHz is placed at the distance of 50 mm to the skin layer (Fig. 3.3). The source is assumed to be inside a matching interface of relative permittivity 40 and a constant conductivity of 1 S/m. The goal is to estimate the amount of reflected power back to the antenna from the blood layer (representing a stroke region in the model). The results of the analysis at several single frequencies up to 5 GHz are presented in the Fig. 3.6 to 3.8.

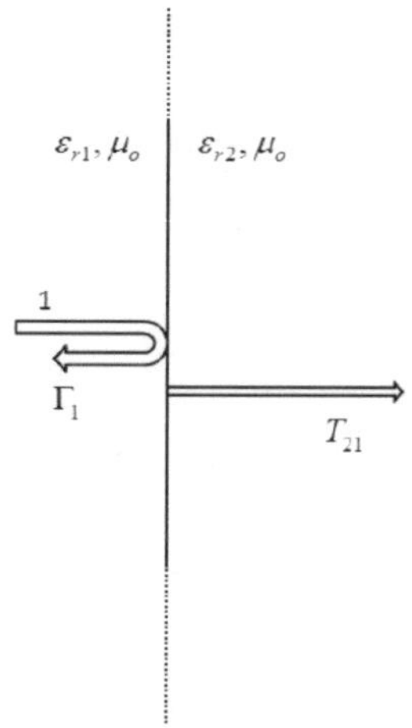

Fig. 3.5: The reflected and transmitted microwave signals at an interface between two medium.

The results show that the amount of power reflected back to the antenna from the blood layer decreases considerably as the frequency increases. It should be emphasized that the presented results serve only as an initial estimation that corresponds to a simple planar head model and many realistic issues are missing in the analysis. Here is a list of some approximations:

1. the model is planar and the real geometrical shape of the head tissues and their curvatures are not included in the model,
2. higher-order diffraction contributions and multiple reflections are neglected mainly due to their anticipated weak contributions compared to the 1st order contributions.
3. the loss and inefficiencies of the different components of the measurement system such as cables and connectors are not taken into account.

In a real scenario the dispersion and attenuation of the real head tissues are expected to be worse at each individual frequency and the diffraction of microwave

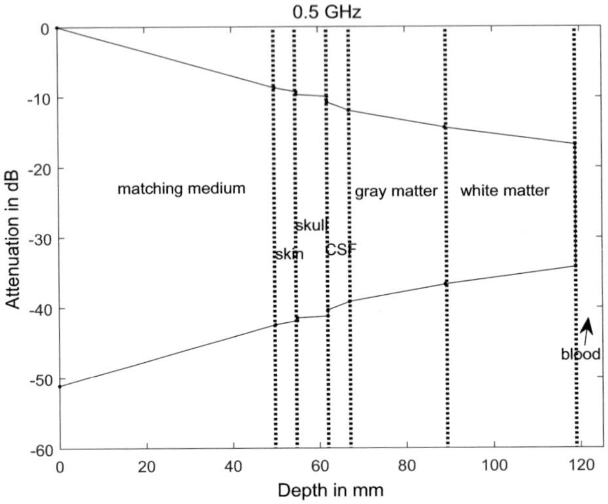

(a)

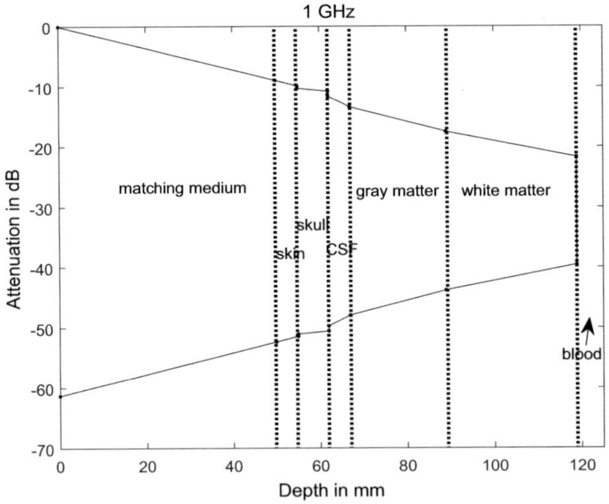

(b)

Fig. 3.6: (a) Attenuation at 0.5 GHz; the reflected power back to the transmitter from the blood layer at 0.5 GHz. (b) Attenuation at 1 GHz; the reflected power back to the transmitter from the blood layer at 1 GHz.

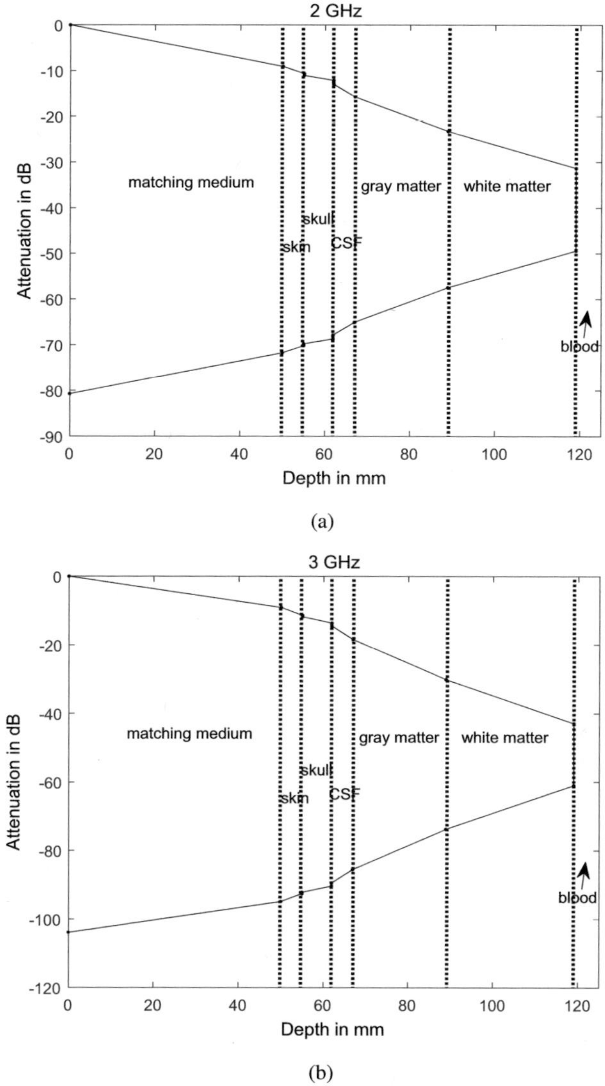

Fig. 3.7: (a) Attenuation at 2 GHz; the reflected power back to the transmitter from the blood layer at 2 GHz. (b) Attenuation result at 3 GHz; the reflected power back to the transmitter from the blood layer at 3 GHz.

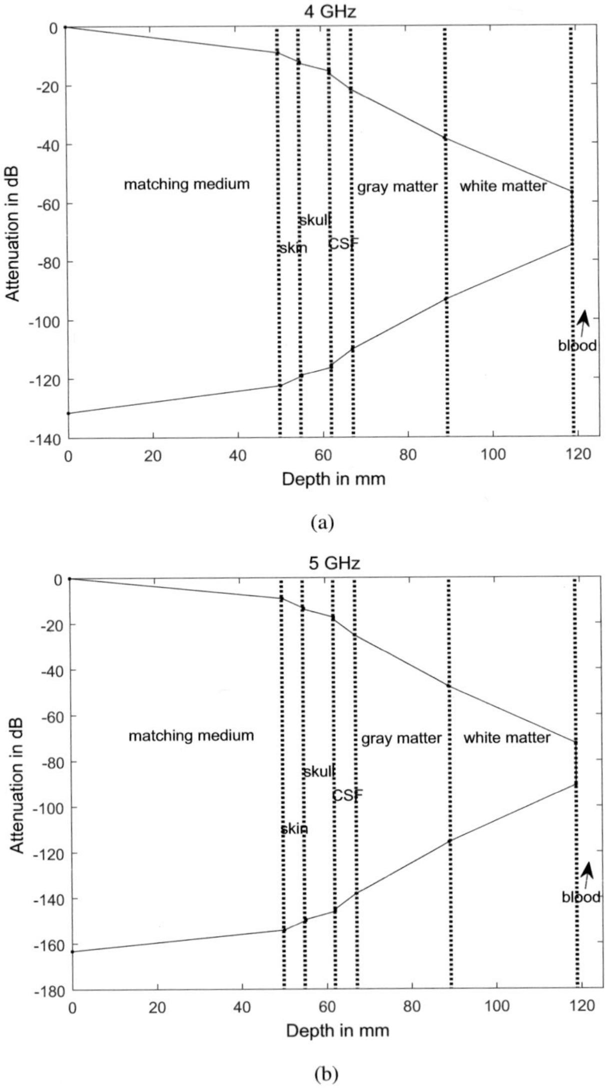

Fig. 3.8: (a) Attenuation at 4 GHz; the reflected power back to the transmitter from the blood layer at 4 GHz. (b) Attenuation result at 5 GHz; the reflected power back to the transmitter from the blood layer at 5 GHz.

signals at the interface of each layer is expected to be far more complicated. Still considering these results low frequencies around 500 MHz are recommended. These frequencies allow deep penetration into the head layers where the stroke might happen (Fig. 3.6 (a)). On the other hand, the best resolution can be achieved at high frequencies due to the small wavelength at such frequencies. However, as conformed by the results of the analysis in this section, the highest frequency is limited due to the higher attenuation of the microwave signals and as a result lower signal to noise ratio (SNR) as the frequency increases. Therefore, for a detection of stroke, a compromise needs to be done between the high resolution and reliable SNR. On the basis of the discussion so far and according to the results in Figs. 3.7 to 3.8, an upper limit of 2 GHz is recommended. Up to 2 GHz the attenuation of the microwave signals seems to be tolerable and it might be possible to detect the stroke with reliable SNR. It has to be emphasized that the construction of efficient and compact antennas with high fractional bandwidths in the frequency range of 0.5 - 2 GHz is a big challenge [32] and [61].

In the following, a numerically realistic 2D head model is imaged in a simulation scenario at 1 GHz.

3.3 Numerical investigation of hemorrhagic stroke detection using microwave tomography

In this section, an anatomically realistic 2D head model extracted from [62] with an artificially embedded hemorrhagic stroke region is simulated in an FDTD solver using 24 ideal point source antennas surrounding the model in a form of a square array. Using a nonlinear iterative image reconstruction algorithm based on Gauss-Newton optimization implemented in C++, the head model is successfully reconstructed after 10 iterations starting from a homogeneous initial guess (blind inversion).

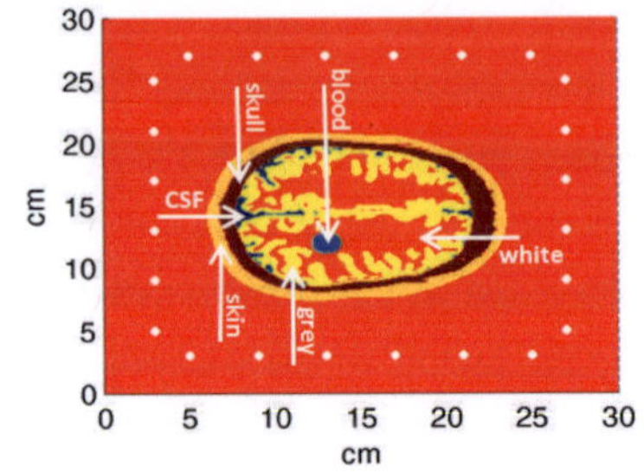

Fig. 3.9: The 2D numerical head model and the point-source array surrounding it; dimension of the array is 24 cm x 24 cm

3.3.1 MRI-derived head model

The MRI-derived head model includes 5 layers: skin, skull, CSF, gray matter and white matter. The dielectric properties of each layer are estimated using the Cole-Cole formula at the single frequency of 1 GHz and are listed in Table 3.2. The imported numerical head model (1 mm resolution) is surrounded by 24 ideal point antennas in a form of a square array (distance between adjacent elements 4 cm) (see Fig. 3.9). An area of stroke (blood) modeled as a circle of radius 8.5 mm is further inserted to the head model. Fig. 3.10 presents a quantitative view of the dielectric properties of the layers (contrast of the tissues) and their corresponding thickness at a cut line passing through the center of the blood circle. The head model of Fig. 3.9 is first simulated in the FDTD software MEEP [52] and following a multistatic scenario 24 x 23 scattered electric fields (referred to E_{meas}) are obtained at 1 GHz.

3.3.2 Imaging algorithm: nonlinear iterative Gauss-Newton

In a MT imaging system, the image reconstruction is essentially based on the comparison between the measured electric fields and the electric fields obtained by the numerical simulation of the measurement system (performed by the so called forward solver). The dielectric properties of the imaging object are retrie-

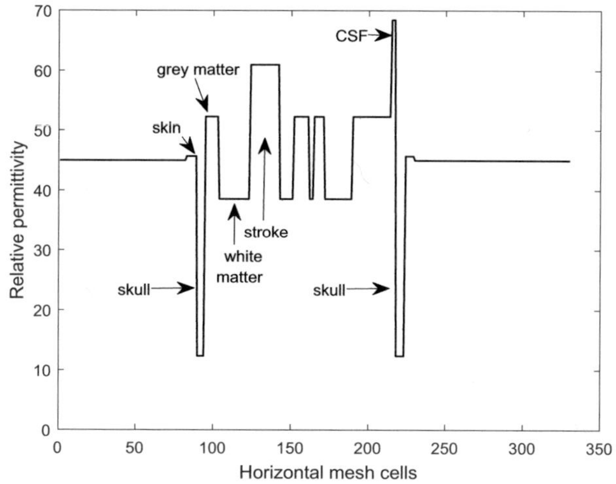

(a)

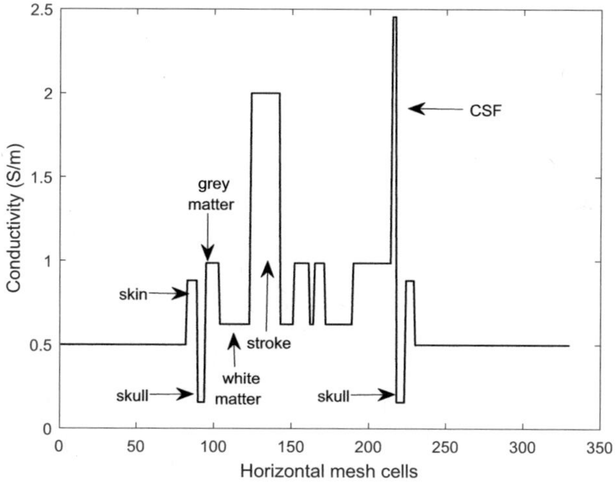

(b)

Fig. 3.10: The relative permittivity and conductivity assigned to the MRI-extracted numerical model at 1 GHz; a horizontal cut at the position of blood (stroke). (a) relative permittivity, (b) conductivity.

Tabelle 3.2: Dielectric characteristics of the numerical head model at 1 GHz

	Relative permittivity	Conductivity (S / m)
skin	45.71	0.88
skull	12.36	0.155
CSF	68.44	2.45
gray matter	52.28	0.98
white matter	38.58	0.62
stroke (blood)	61	2
matching medium	45	0.5

ved by minimizing the discrepancies between the scattered electric fields of the numerical model E_{sim} and the measured scattered electric fields E_{meas} obtained after calibration [22] and [53]. This minimization can be formulated as:

$$min \Longrightarrow ||E_{meas} - E_{sim}||^2 \tag{3.5}$$

Following an iterative procedure based on a Gauss-Newton optimization, the complex permittivity of each mesh cell of the model will be updated in a way to lead to the minimization of the discrepancy between the measured and simulated scattered electric fields in equation (3.5). The new complex permittivity at the end of each iteration will be estimated as:

$$\varepsilon_{n+1} = \varepsilon_n + \Delta\varepsilon \tag{3.6}$$

ε_n is the complex relative permittivity at the nth iteration. The increment in the real part and the imaginary parts of ε are estimated in every other iterations successively using:

$$\Delta\varepsilon = (J^T J + \lambda I)^{-1} J^T (E_{meas.} - E_{sim.}) \tag{3.7}$$

J is the jacobian (sensitivity) matrix and in this research it is evaluated numerically using the finite difference method.

$$J_{ij} = \frac{\delta\, E_{sim}}{\delta \varepsilon_{ij}} = \frac{E_{sim}(\varepsilon_{ij} + h) - E_{sim}(\varepsilon_{ij})}{h} \tag{3.8}$$

where h is set to $\frac{\varepsilon_{ij}}{100}$. i and j refer to the each of the mesh cells in the simulation domain. Therefore it takes one simulation of the forward solver per mesh cell. I is the identity matrix and the operator T refers to conjugate transpose of the matrix.

Furthermore, since the inverse problem is severely ill-posed, a regularization procedure is needed to stabilize the image reconstruction procedure. Tikhonov regularization [22] is one efficient stabilizing technique. In (3.7), λ is the Tikhonov regularization factor and is estimated according to:

$$\lambda = \alpha[\frac{1}{N}\sum_{i=1}^{N} J^T J(i,i)][err_E]^2 \tag{3.9}$$

α adjusts the magnitude of the regularization and is chosen empirically according to the convergence of the reconstruction process. (3.9) involves further the trace of the matrix JJ^T and the relative mean square error of the simulated and measured scattered fields.

The imaging procedure can be summarized as follows (see Fig. 3.11):

- In the reconstruction procedure, no priori information [18] about the brain model (shape of the layers or the dielectric properties) is assumed and therefore as the initial guess (first iteration) all the 8100 mesh cells (3 mesh cells per 1 centimeter that is: $30 \times 3 \times 30 \times 3 = 8100$ mesh cells) are assumed to have the dielectric properties of the background (see Table 3.2). The complex permittivity of the background matching medium is approximated as the weighted average complex permittivity of all the head layers at 1 GHz (Fig. 3.12)).

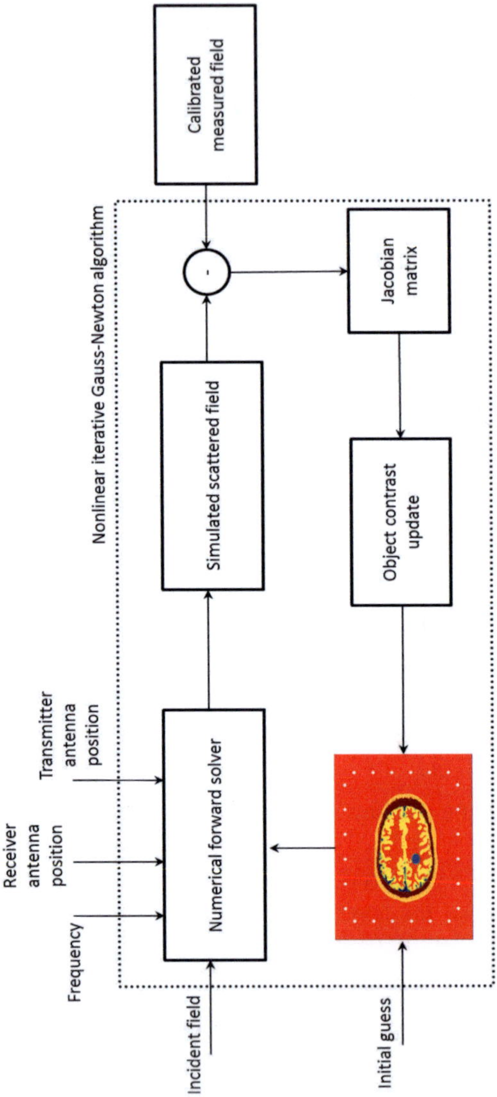

Fig. 3.11: An overview of the nonlinear iterative image reconstruction algorithm used for imaging.

- With the assumed dielectric distribution, the scattered electric fields are simulated (E_{sim}) and the jacobian matrix is estimated according to (3.8).
- The complex permittivity map is afterwards updated according to (3.7) and therefore following (3.6) a new distribution of the complex permittivity is obtained. Going to the previous step of determining the new simulated electric field corresponding to the new permittivity profile, the process is iteratively repeated until the convergence criteria is relaxed (here: until the new reconstructed permittivity and conductivity is not significantly different from the previous iteration).

3.3.3 Simulated imaging results at 1 GHz

The reconstructed images of the relative permittivity and conductivity at the frequency of 1 GHz after the first iteration are shown in Fig. 3.13a and 3.13b. It is observed that starting from a homogeneous distribution equal to background permittivity and conductivity without any prior information about the head model, right after the first iteration the relative shape of the skull, gray matter, white matter and stroke regions are reconstructed and the left and right side of the brain are clearly distinguished in the permittivity map (Fig. 3.13a) (only the CSF layer is hard to realize mostly due to its very small thickness). Above all, the stroke region is clearly detected right after the first iteration. After the 10th iteration, it is further possible to realize the skin layer and an acceptable shape reconstruction, the permittivity and conductivity of the layers also compare to actual values in Table 3.2 (Fig. 3.13 (b)). The root mean square errors of the reconstructions after each iteration are listed in Table 3.3. In Fig. 3.14 the original dielectric properties of the tissues and the reconstructed values after the 10th iteration are compared along a line passing through the center of the blood circle.
These results motivate the application of microwave imaging (tomographic approach) for the detection of stroke in a human head. However, when it comes to the implementation of an imaging system for head imaging, many practical is-

sues have to be carefully considered. Very determining is the design of efficient antenna structures for effective illumination of the imaging object and capturing the scattered signals at different observation points around the IO. The main focus of the research in this dissertation is proposing antenna structures for different microwave imaging approaches and introducing criteria for the evaluation of the performance of such antennas. It will be discussed that each imaging modality demands a different specification of the antenna and although an antenna structure might work efficiently for one microwave imaging technology, it can present a poor performance in another.

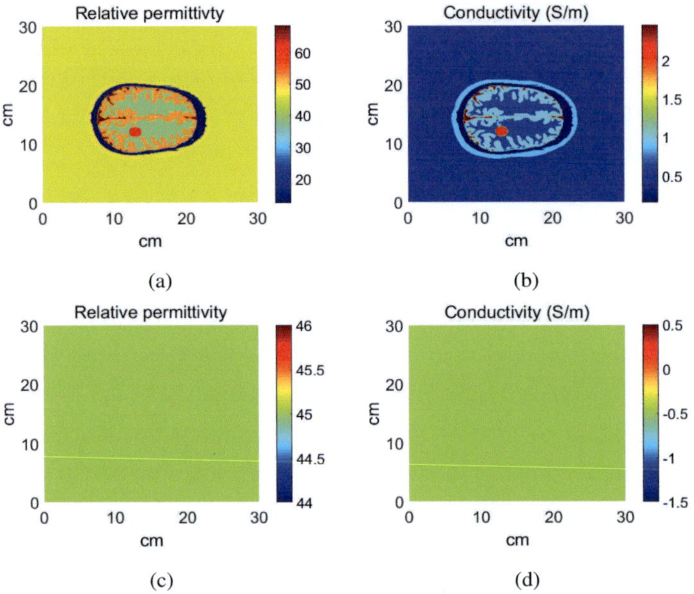

Fig. 3.12: 1st column: relative permittivity; 2nd column: conductivity at 1 GHz; (a) and (b) the original map of the relative permittivity and conductivity of the imported numerical head model; (c) and (d) the initial guess at the begin of the iterations.

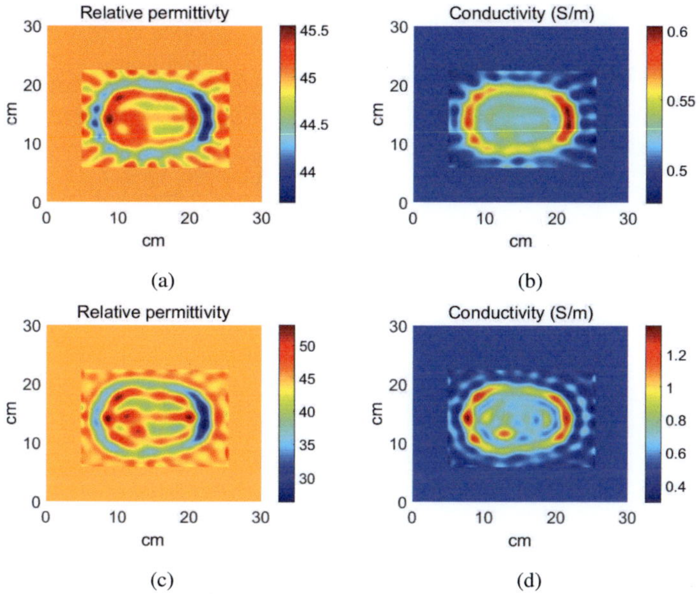

Fig. 3.13: 1st column: relative permittivity; 2nd column: conductivity at 1 GHz; (a) and (b) the reconstructed images after the 1st iteration; (c) and (d) the reconstructed images after the 10th iteration.

Tabelle 3.3: The root mean square error (RMSE) after each iteration

Iteration number	RMSE
1	0.432643
2	0.35533
3	0.291244
4	0.23823
5	0.194454
6	0.158381
7	0.128715
8	0.104374
9	0.0844536
10	0.0682052

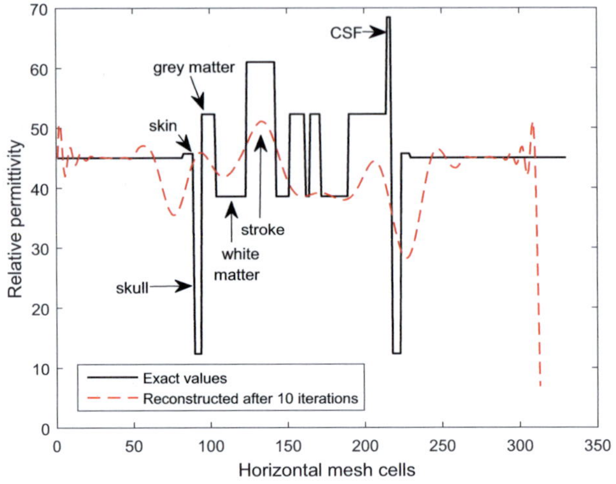

(a)

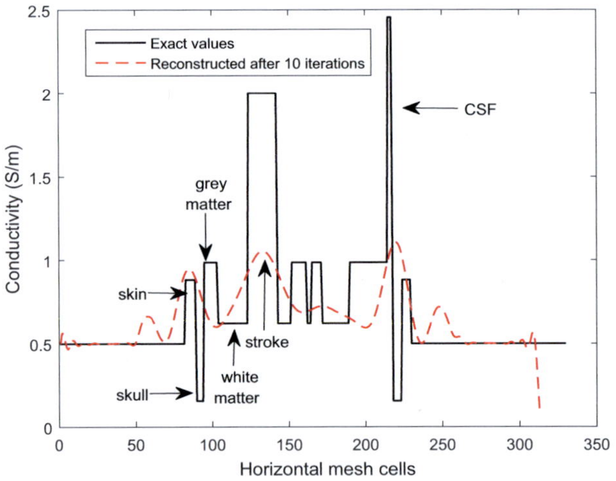

(b)

Fig. 3.14: The reconstructed relative permittivity and conductivity at 1 GHz compared to the exact values originally assigned to the mesh cells; a horizontal cut at the position of stroke.

4 Efficient antenna for full-wave 3D microwave tomography

In microwave tomography (MT), low-power signals are transmitted toward the imaging object (IO) by an array of antennas surrounding the IO enabling a 3D illumination. Signals scattered in different directions are captured by receive antennas and the distribution of the dielectric properties of the IO is then reconstructed using nonlinear inverse scattering approaches.
The degree of success of the imaging in MT depends to a high extent on the accuracy of the numerical model of the measurement setup in the forward solver. Recently, following the advances in microwave technology and image reconstruction techniques, 3D microwave tomography has been exploited worldwide for practical medical applications [78] and [19]. In this chapter, the antenna requirements for full-wave 3D microwave tomography imaging are discussed. An efficient antenna structure is proposed for this imaging method. The performance of the proposed antenna is further compared to the so far most widely used antenna for this application.

4.1 Antenna requirement for full-wave 3D microwave tomography

In full-wave 3D microwave tomography the IO is surrounded by a 3D antenna array (mostly cylindrical array configuration as shown in Fig. 4.1). In the imaging procedure using nonlinear inverse scattering approaches, the accuracy of the numerical simulation of the measurement system is a major challenge. Ideally, the numerical simulation has to represent the measurement setup as exactly as possible. This would lead to the least artifact and clutter in the final reconstructed imaging results. However, a more realistic numerical simulation means taking more details of the measurement system into account (e.g. exact antenna structure) and this would naturally impose more computational load to the system in each iteration. Antennas are therefore known to directly influence the ultimate accuracy of the imaging system [12] and [1].

To avoid the complexity of the numerical solver model, the antenna structure has to be as simple as possible so that modeling the antenna numerically in the forward solver would impose little extra computational cost on the numerical solver. Furthermore, since multi-frequency or UWB imaging offers several invaluable advantages over mono-frequency approaches, the optimum antenna element should maintain a stable characteristic over a large bandwidth.

The most widely used antennas for microwave tomography so far are monopoles and dipoles [76]. Although these antennas offer simplicity in terms of forward solver modeling, they are associated with some serious inefficiencies. The omnidirectional radiation of these antennas increases the sensitivity of the imaging system to the environmental interference and therefore degrades the reconstruction results. The resonance antennas are mostly utilized inside lossy interface mediums in order to increase the bandwidth and reduce the background effect, however this simultaneously leads to the decreased sensitivity of the imaging system to the desired signals. Therefore, an alternative simple structure broadband element is desired for application in full-wave 3D microwave tomography.

In this section, a modified Bowtie antenna is proposed for 3D full-wave microwave tomography. The proposed antenna is compared to a simple monopole structure widely used in the imaging systems based on 3D microwave tomography. The two antenna structures are compared regarding the important requirements for the imaging procedure of 3D microwave tomography; i.e. the coupled power inside an example IO and the computational load.

In the overall design procedure the following antenna specification are set as ultimate goals:

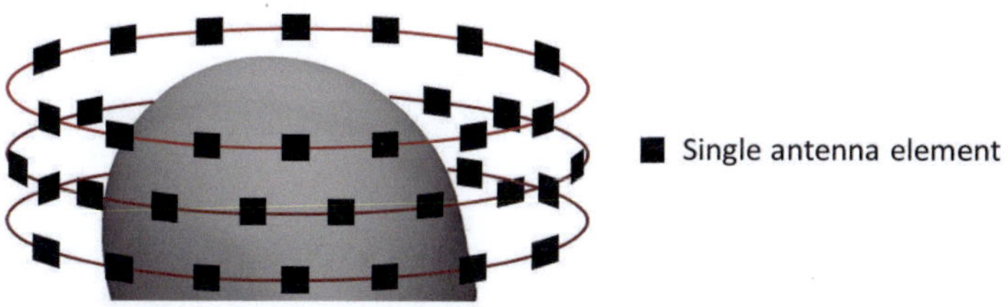

Fig. 4.1: Antenna array surrounding an imaging object in full-wave 3D microwave tomography enabling a 3D illumination of the IO.

1. The optimum antenna should be compact allowing for a large number of elements in the array.
2. The structure of the antenna should offer simplicity when it comes to modeling in the numerical forward solver.
3. A broadband performance covering a lower spectrum is desired to enable deep penetration and high resolution.

4.2 Description of the modified Bowtie Antenna

As a starting point, the idea was to modify the antenna structure previously proposed in [32] in order to enhance the performance of the antenna regarding the operational bandwidth and further to simplify the structure of the antenna to make it a more suitable option in 3D microwave tomography.
The antenna is designed to operate inside a bio-compatible matching liquid composed of Ethanol and water (weight ratio of 1:1) (at 1 GHz : $\varepsilon_r = 42, \sigma = 0.5S/m$). The measured dielectric properties of pure water, ethanol and the 50% solution are presented in Fig. 4.2 to 4.4. The measured dielectric properties of the ethanol-water solution are imported and used during the simulation and optimization of the antenna in CST Microwave Studio.

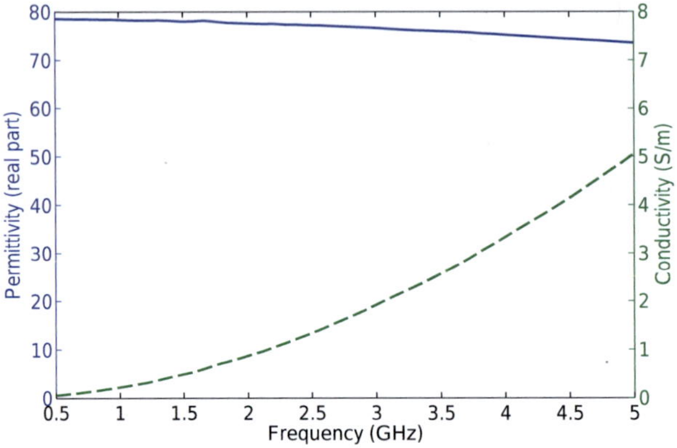

Fig. 4.2: Dielectric properties of pure water; solid line: relative permittivity, dashed line: conductivity.

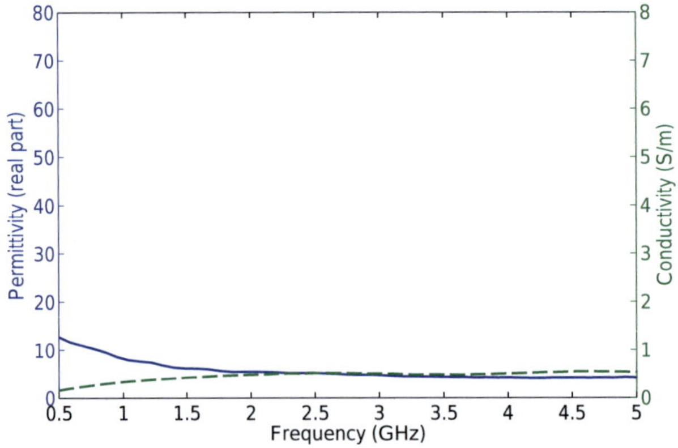

Fig. 4.3: Dielectric properties of pure ethanol; solid line: relative permittivity, dashed line: conductivity.

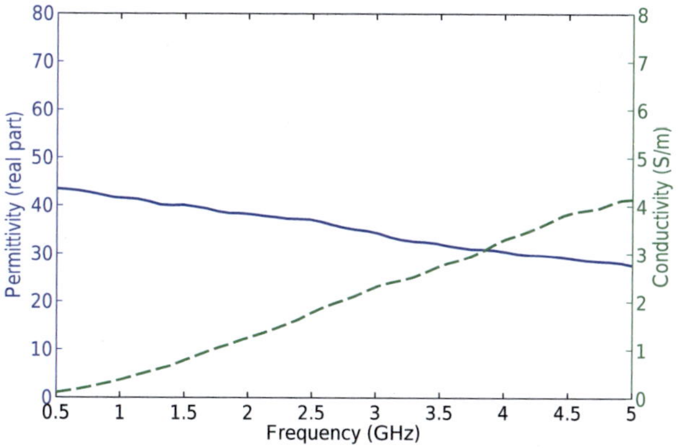

Fig. 4.4: Dielectric properties of 50% water-ethanol solution; solid line: relative permittivity, dashed line: conductivity.

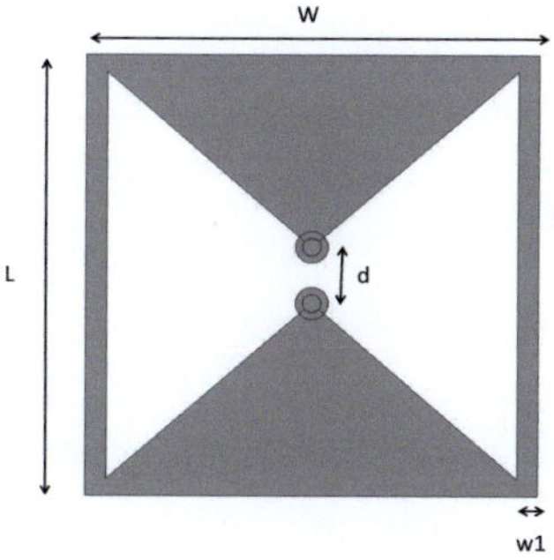

Fig. 4.5: The proposed antenna structure with a straight connection between the two arms of the Bowtie.

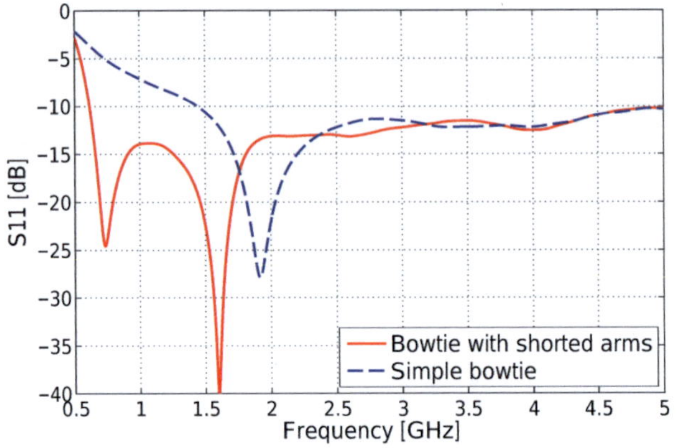

Fig. 4.6: Reflection coefficient of a model with discrete feeding with and without short-connection between the arms of the Bow-tie.

The layout of the proposed Bowtie antenna is shown in Fig. 4.5. In this layout, the two arms of the conventional Bowtie antenna are connected via straight strips placed on the upper side of the substrate. The idea is to add inductive strips to compensate for the capacitive nature of the antenna and therefore the lower cut-off frequency can be decreased. The impact of the strip connection between the arms on the antenna matching is being investigated by simulating the same antenna (with discrete port feeding) with and without the connections (the optimal width of the shorting strips is found to be w1=1 mm). The matching of the antenna in the two configurations is compared in Fig. 4.6 which clearly shows the considerable improvement in the bandwidth extension upon using the strips. It is observed that after short-connecting the two arms of a conventional Bowtie antenna, it is possible to cover low frequencies below 1 GHz without any need to enlarge the dimension of the antenna (normally, the lowest frequency of operation is limited by the physical dimension of the antenna). Meanwhile, it is also observed that the reflection coefficient of the antenna at higher frequencies is still quite acceptable.

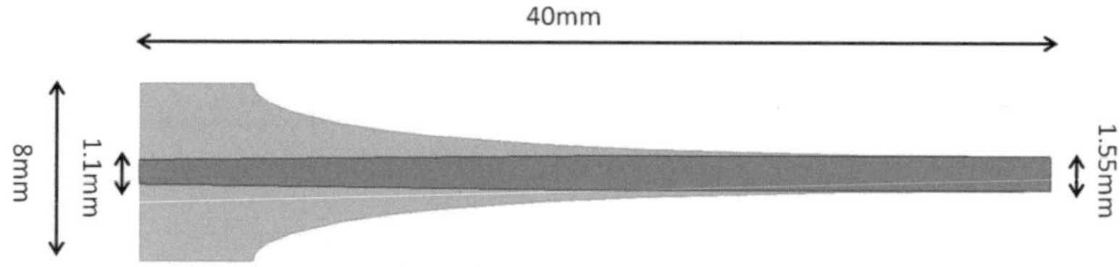

Fig. 4.7: The balun structure with the optimized dimension simulated in CST microwave studio.

To ease the modeling of the antenna element in the 3D numerical forward solver, we are specially interested in an antenna with symmetric radiation resembling the radiation of an ideally fed antenna so that there would be no need to model the feeding part and as a result to avoid the additional computational cost associated with the feeding.

To achieve this goal, instead of the unbalanced coaxial cable feeding of the previous antenna design in [32], the feeding via a balun is recommended. The optimized balun in Fig. 4.7 is fabricated on a Rogers 6010 substrate ($\varepsilon_r = 10.2$ and thickness of 1.27 mm). The antenna was optimized in CST microwave studio to maintain a directive radiation from below 1 GHz to nearly 3 GHz. After optimization, with the values of W and L set to 22 mm (Fig. 4.5), the spacing d is set to 2.8 mm after optimization. The radiating element is fabricated on a Rogers 5880 substrate ($\varepsilon_r = 2.2$ and thickness of 1.5 mm). The fabricated antenna is shown in Fig. 4.8.

To evaluate the effectiveness of the balun, the performance of the Bowtie antenna using two feeding structures: ideal discrete port and feeding via balun has been investigated via simulations. The normalized E-field radiated from the antenna in each case is displayed in Fig. 4.9. It can be seen that the radiated E-field of the antenna with the balun structure agrees to that of the ideal discrete port feeding. This means that the Bowtie antenna fed by the balun structure can be efficiently modeled in the 3D numerical forward solver by only the radiating element and still the radiated E-field would highly resemble that of the actual antenna.

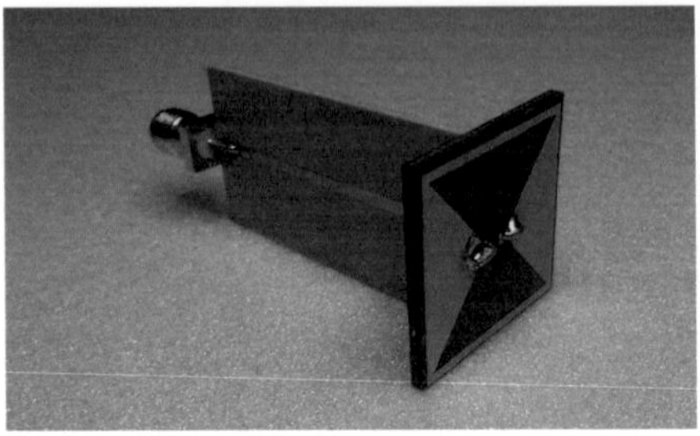

Fig. 4.8: The fabricated antenna with the balun feeding.

4.3 Measurement of the modified Bowtie Antenna

The Bowtie antenna with the previously optimized parameters fed through a balun is afterwards fabricated (see Fig. 4.8) and characterized experimentally. The antenna is designed so that the radiating part of the antenna has to be directly in contact to a high-permittivity medium (either inside a maching liquid or directly on tissue-mimicking phantom). Therefore to simulate a real scenario, the fabricated antenna is packed in a Styrofoam box to assist the radiation pattern measurement The antenna is afterwards immersed in 50% ethanol-water solution for the reflectivity and radiation pattern measurements.

The simulated and measured reflection coefficient results are presented in Fig. 4.10. As can be seen, the lowest operational frequency of the antenna is around 0.8 GHz and the reflection coefficient stays below -10 dB up to around 5 GHz. However,as mentioned before, it was observed during simulations that above 3 GHz the main radiation beam of the antenna splits in two directions (Fig.4.11 to 4.12). Therefore, the operational bandwidth of the antenna is from 0.8 to 3 GHz. To measure the radiation pattern of the antenna immersed in the ethanol-water solution, the near field measurement setup explained in [34] was used and the antenna packed in a styrofoam box was inserted into the matching liquid solution (Fig. 4.13). In the near-field measurement setup, the radiated field inside the

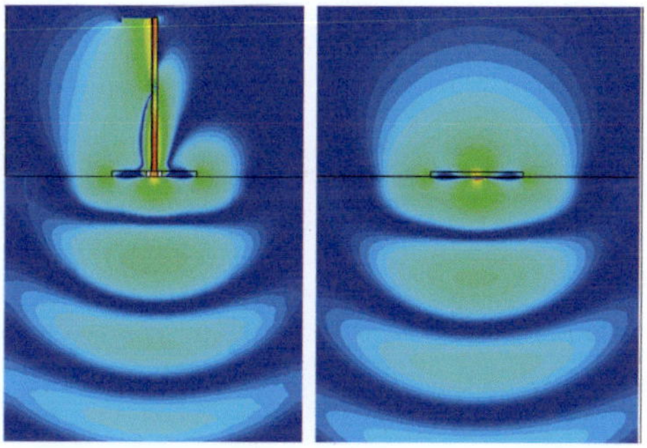

(a)

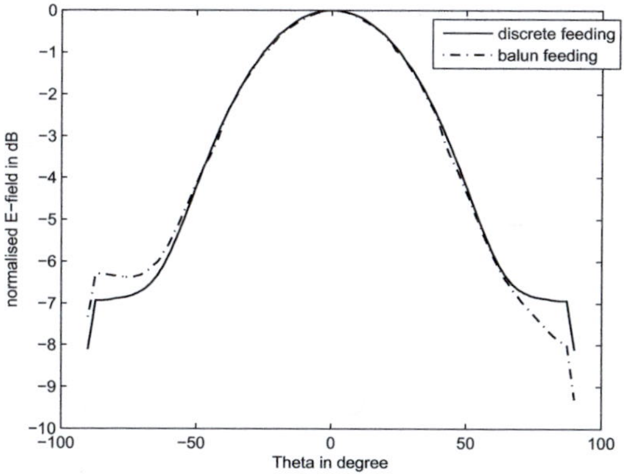

(b)

Fig. 4.9: Comparison of the normalized E-field pattern at 1.5 GHz. (a) Tapered microstrip balun (left) and Ideally symmetric discrete port feeding (right); (b) Normalized E-field at the distance of 30 mm to the antenna.

matching liquid is scanned in a planar-rectangular area. The far field pattern is obtained afterwards using the near field to far field transformation [34].

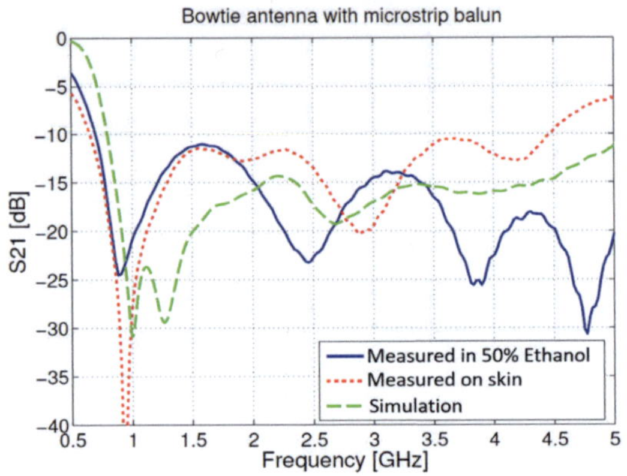

Fig. 4.10: The reflection coefficient of the Bowtie antenna; simulation and measurement results.

The results of the measured antenna radiation characteristics for vertical and horizontal polarizations are displayed in Fig. 4.14. The radiation pattern measured for horizontal polarization is directive and ideally symmetric. The coupling between the arms of the Bowtie and the current flowing down the feeding in the vertical polarization is being minimized using the balun structure.

So far, a compact broadband Bowtie antenna operating from 0.8 to 3 GHz is proposed. The miniaturization technique of connecting the two arms of the Bowtie antenna, enabled the extension of the operational bandwidth to frequencies lower than 1 GHz. Furthermore, the radiation of the antenna was shown to be independent of its balun feeding network. This would be a great advantage for the application in 3D microwave tomography, since the antenna can be fully represented only by its radiation part and therefore, a lot of computational time can be saved.

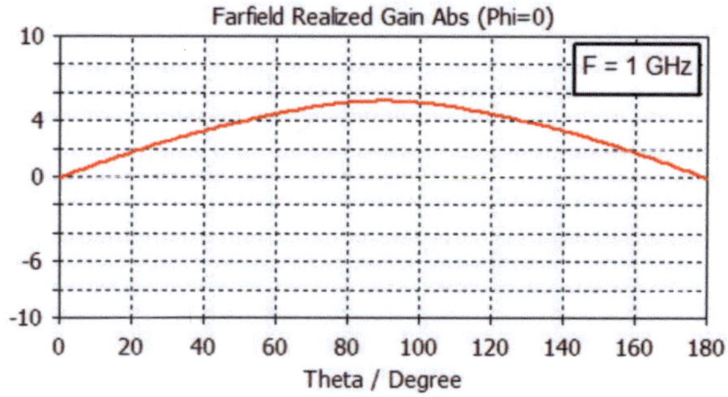

(a)

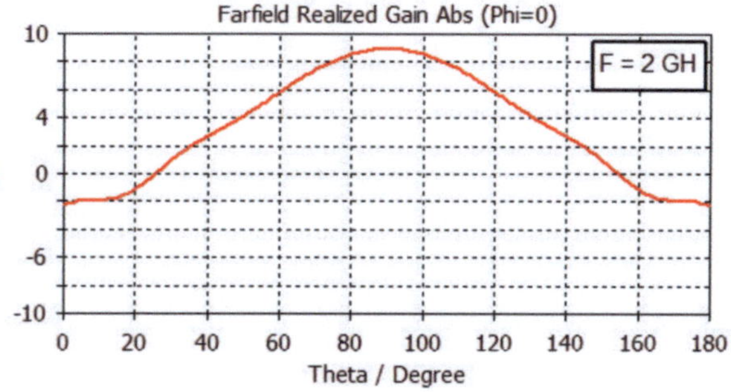

(b)

Fig. 4.11: Simulated far-field radiation pattern of the modified Bowtie antenna- I.

4.4 The modified Bowtie antenna compared to a conventional monopole antenna

As stated before, simple monopole antennas are most commonly used in 3D microwave tomography systems for medical applications [76], [72] and [81]. The antennas are originally resonance elements but their bandwidth increases when immersed in lossy matching interfaces.

The main advantage of using monopole antennas for full-wave 3D microwave tomography systems is the ease of the modeling of the antenna in the numerical 3D forward solver and the minimum computational load it composes to the imaging algorithms compared to the other more complicated antenna structures.

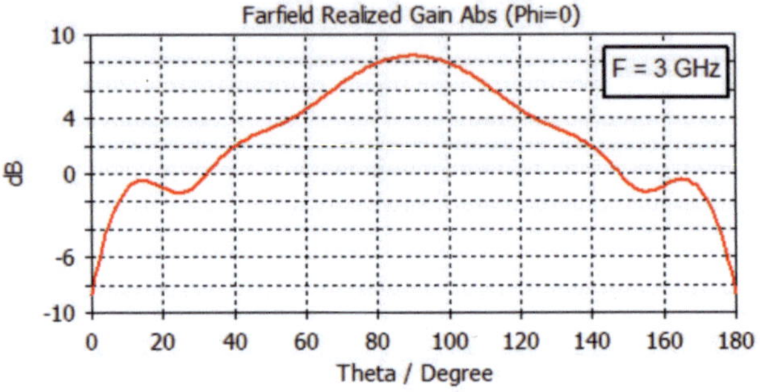

(a)

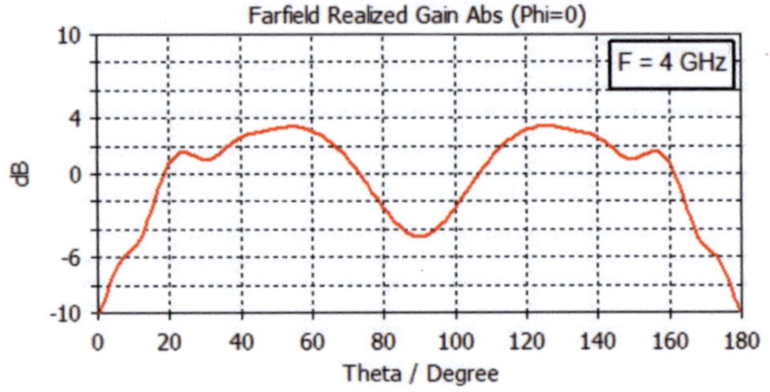

(b)

Fig. 4.12: Simulated far-field radiation pattern of the modified Bowtie antenna- II.

The major drawback of the antenna, however, is its low efficiency in radiating the EM signals toward the object. This is mainly due to the omnidirectional radiation pattern of the antenna. The imaging systems implementing monopole antenna arrays are especially vulnerable to interference signals from the surroundings.

In this section, the previously developed modified Bowtie antenna is compared to a conventional monopole antenna regarding some important criteria for 3D microwave tomography systems; namely simulation time and the coupled power into an IO. As an example scenario, both antennas are evaluated and compared for the specific application of head imaging.

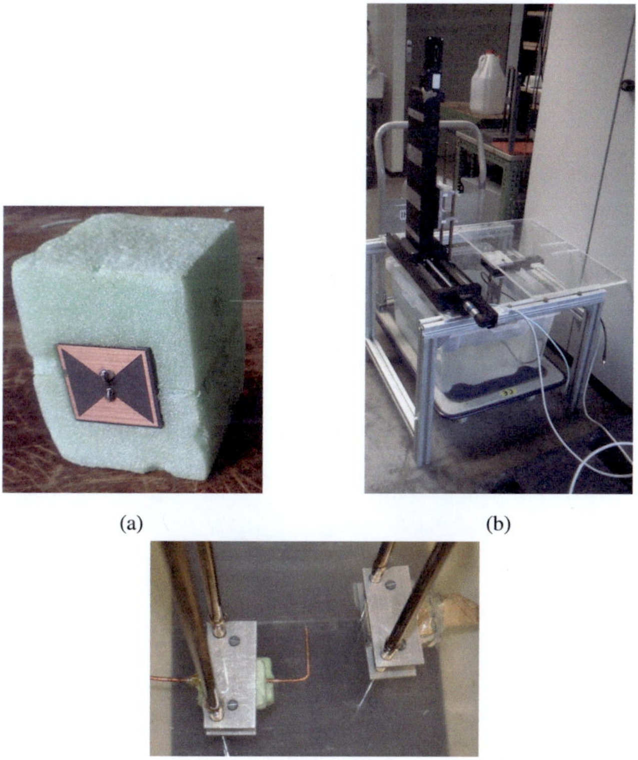

(a) (b)

(c)

Fig. 4.13: Near field measurement of the Bowtie antenna. (a) the antenna wrapped in Styrofoam; (b) a view of the near-field measurement system; (c) the measurement probe for capturing the near-field radiation of the Bowtie antenna.

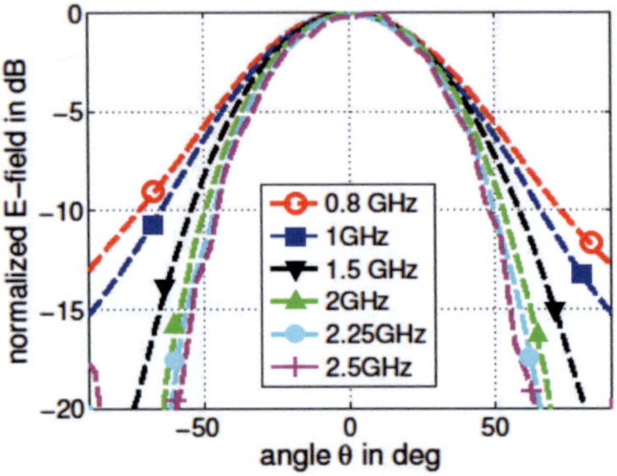

(a) horizontal polarization

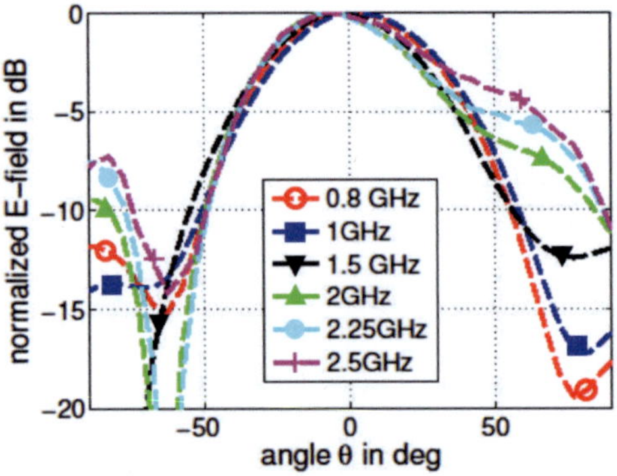

(b) vertical polarization

Fig. 4.14: The normalized E-field radiated by the Bowtie antenna; measurement results.

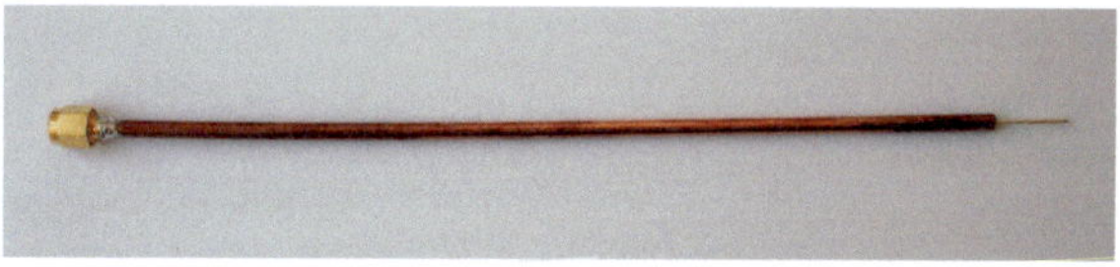

(a)

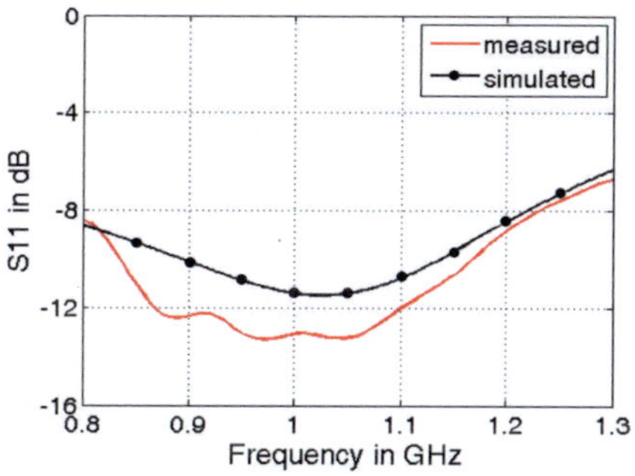

(b)

Fig. 4.15: The monopole antenna and its reflection coefficient.

4.4.1 Monopole antenna for microwave medical imaging

Monopole antenna can be simply realized by exposing a quarter of wavelength of a coaxial cable inner conductor in a medium. This kind of antenna is poorly behaved in lossless medium such as air, because it excites currents on the outer conductor. However, its behavior changes when it is immersed inside a lossy medium, because unwanted currents are attenuated and its bandwidth increases. The fabricated monopole antenna for head imaging is shown in Fig. 4.15 (a). The total length is 20.6 cm, while the length of the active part is 1.6 cm. The diameter of inner and outer conductors are 0.9 mm and 3.581 mm respectively. The S11 parameter was measured while the antenna was immersed in the 50%

ethanol-water solution. As can be seen in Fig. 4.15 (b), the antenna is matched below -8 dB in a frequency range of 0.8 - 1.2 GHz. It has to be mentioned that although the monopole antenna presents some broadband characteristic when immersed in the lossy interface of ethanol-water solution, still its bandwidth is quite small compared to the previously proposed modified Bowtie antenna (Fig. 4.10).

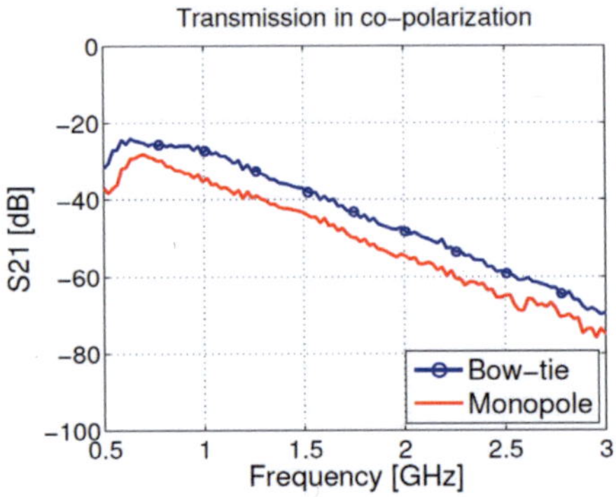

Fig. 4.16: The measured transmission of the Monopole and Bowtie antennas compared in co-polarization with respect to the receiving probe in the near-field measurement system.

The two antennas are further compared regarding the transmission capabilities when used in the near field measurement system of Fig. 4.13 in co-polarization configuration with respect to the measurement probe. The result of the comparison is shown in Fig. 4.16. It is observed that the Bowtie antenna transmits approximately 10 dB more power to the measurement probe compared to the monopole antenna in the whole frequency range.

In the following, the two antenna structures are compared regarding their capabilities of directing microwave power into an IO and their associated simulation time (computational time) in a 3D solver.

4.4.2 Comparison regarding the coupled power into a multilayer head model

To compare the modified Bowtie antenna to the simple monopole antenna, a scenario is simulated in CST microwave studio. In two separate simulations, each antenna element is positioned at a constant distance (60 mm) to a cylindrical multilayer head model having four dispersive layers. The biggest dimension of the head model is 140 mm. Antennas are placed inside a matching medium equivalent to 50% water-ethanol solution.

With the same setup in the two simulations, the absolute value of the power coupled into the head phantom is compared for the two antennas at four frequencies from 0.5 to 2 GHz (these frequencies were recommended to be the optimal range for head imaging in the previous chapter).

The simulated coupled power levels into the head model from the monopole antenna at four different frequencies are shown in Fig. 4.17. It is observed that the amount of absolute power fades as the frequency increases. This is because the monopole antenna was previously shown to be best matched in a narrow bandwidth around 1 GHz. Furthermore, as expected it is clearly observed that the monopole antenna has no priority in the direction of radiation because of its omnidirectional radiation pattern. This is regarded as one major disadvantage of the monopole antenna for medical imaging applications. It increases the sensitivity of the imaging system to the interference signals from the surrounding of the imaging system and therefore degrades the overall signal to noise ratio of the imaging. Therefore, in case of small imaging tanks, the reflections from the boundaries can not be ignored and they have to be taken into account in the 3D numerical representation of the imaging system and indeed in the imaging algorithms. This would enhance the computational load of the imaging algorithms significantly.

As for the second simulation, the monopole antenna is replaced by the modified Bowtie antenna and the coupled power from the antenna to the multilayer head model is once again estimated. The absolute coupled power at four frequencies from 0.5 to 2 GHz are represented in Fig. 4.18 and they can be directly compared to the corresponding figures of the monopole antenna in Fig. 4.17.

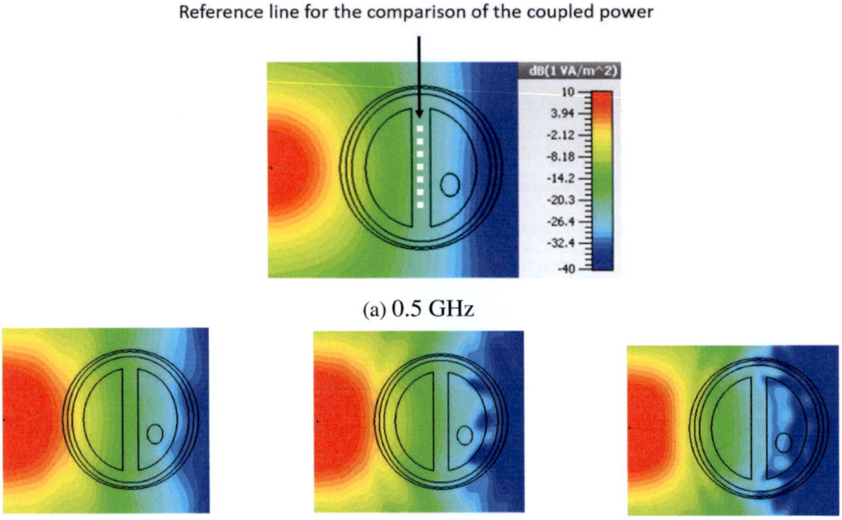

(a) 0.5 GHz

(b) 1 GHz

(c) 1.5 GHz

(d) 2 GHz

Fig. 4.17: The simulated coupled power from the monopole antenna into a multilayer head model at different frequencies.

For a fair and more clear comparison of the coupled power into the multilayer head model in each of the two CST simulations, the absolute values of the coupled power are extracted at a reference line in the middle of the head model (see Fig. 4.17 (a) and 4.18 (a)). The corresponding curves for the monopole and the Bowtie antennas at different frequencies are compared in Fig. 4.19.
As observed in the figure, at all the frequencies the Bowtie antenna directs more power into the head model. The highest power corresponding to the monopole antenna is radiated at 1 GHz and is approximately 8 dB lower than the radia-

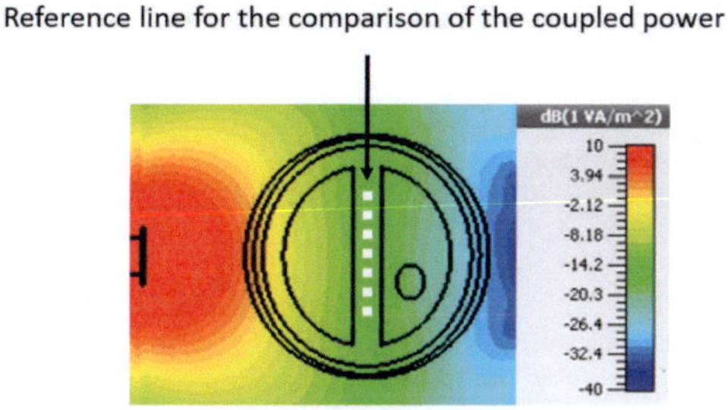

(a) 0.5 GHz

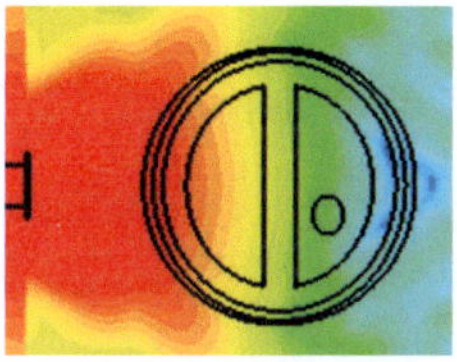

(b) 1 GHz

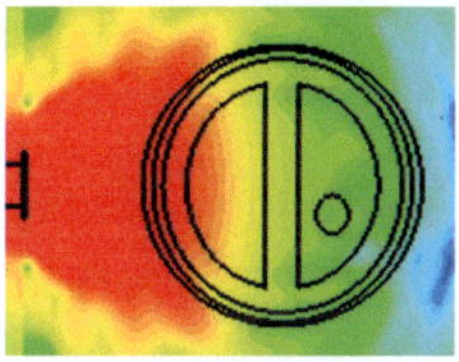

(c) 1.5 GHz

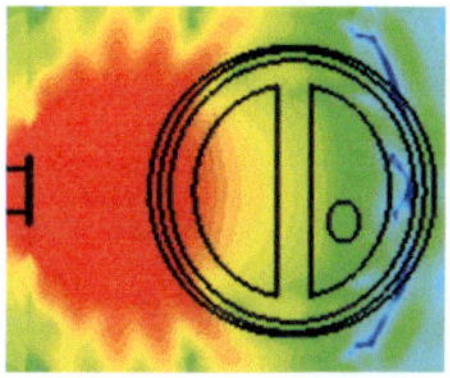

(d) 2 GHz

Fig. 4.18: The simulated coupled power from the Bowtie antenna into a multilayer head model at different frequencies.

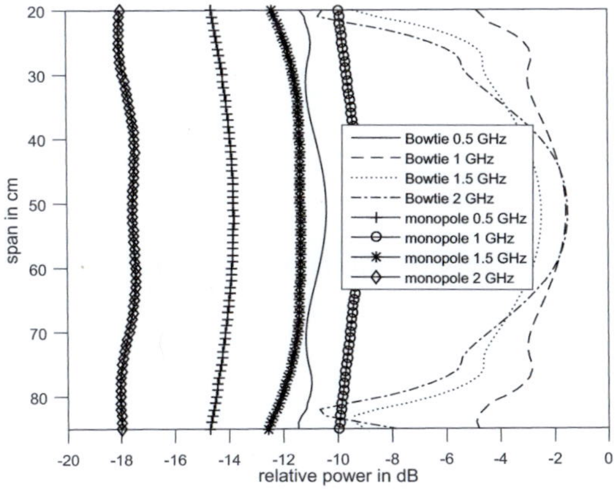

Fig. 4.19: Coupled power to the head model at a reference line in the middle of the head (Fig. 4.18 (a) and 4.18 (a))- comparison of monopole to Bowtie antenna

ted power at the same frequency by the Bowtie antenna in the main radiation direction.

4.4.3 Comparison regarding the computational time

As discussed previously, in full-wave 3D microwave tomography, the measurement system is numerically simulated in the 3D forward solver. Although including more details in the numerical modeling of the measurement system increases the reliability and accuracy of the image reconstruction, it slows down the imaging process by composing more computational load to the imaging algorithms.

Therefore, so far monopole antennas benefiting from their simple structure have been one major choice in the 3D microwave tomography systems for medical applications. In fact, there has been a trade off between the complexity of the imaging system and the efficiency of the antenna element in terms of directing the radiation power into the imaging object and the sensitivity to the weak scattered signals from the targets deep inside the IO ([76], [72] and [81]).

As shown in the previous section, the Bowtie antenna having a larger bandwidth and a more directive radiation pattern, outperforms the simple monopole antenna in terms of the coupled power into an IO. However, the choice of the optimum antenna for 3D microwave tomography depends to a high extent on the resulting complexity of the modeling of the antenna in the numerical solver and the tolerable computational time.

At the beginning of the chapter it was shown that in the simulation of the modified Bowtie antenna, the radiation remains unchanged if the balun feeding is replaced with ideal discrete port feeding. This means that in the 3D numerical modeling of the measurement system, one is allowed to replace the balun feeding with an ideal port feeding to the radiating Bowtie and the radiation of the antenna remains unchanged. This is expected to lead to some decrease of the computational time.

Tabelle 4.1: Monopole antenna and modified Bowtie antenna compared regarding the computational time

antenna	computational time
modified Bowtie with balun feeding	19134 seconds
modified Bowtie with discrete port feeding	5256 seconds
monopole	2151 seconds

To comment on the complexity of the Bowtie and monopole antennas regarding the exposed computational time, the simulation time of the antennas illuminating the multilayer head model in the previous simulation scenario for estimating the coupled power is listed in Table 4.1. In this Table the least computational time corresponds to the monopole antenna illuminating the head model. On the other hand, the complete numerical modeling of the Bowtie antenna with its balun feeding leads to the longest simulation time. However,the required simulation time of the Bowtie antenna drops significantly when the balun feeding is replaced with an ideal discrete port feeding.

Although the computational time associated with the monopole antenna is still less than half of the Bowtie antenna without modeling the balun, this less computational time was in this section shown to be at the expense of the poor radiation of the antenna toward the IO and its high sensitivity to interfering signals from the surrounding objects.

As a result, a compromise needs to be made between the simplicity of the measurement system and the efficiency and reliability of the imaging results. The monopole antenna might work well for simple imaging scenarios when the contrast between the target and the surrounding tissues is high (e.g. cancer detection in high-adipose breast tissues). However, in case of more complex IOs when only a poor backscattered signal from the target is expected (e.g. head imaging for the detection of stroke) a more efficient antenna element is required to enable deep illumination of the object and detection of the smallest scattered signals with a high sensitivity.

5 Efficient antenna for synthetic 3D microwave tomography

In full-wave 3D microwave tomography approach, although fast data acquisition remains an important issue, the major bottleneck is that of the forward solver modeling of the imaging system and the computational load imposed to the inverse solver as a result of the whole system modeling required in 3D imaging [12]. Specially for some relatively large target applications such as stroke detection, the size of the 3D model will be a real obstacle that hinders the efficiency of the imaging.

Synthetic 3D microwave tomography, on the other hand, is referred to an imaging approach in which the object is scanned in several horizontal layers using a 2D antenna array. The scattered signals in each layer are processed using 2D nonlinear iterative image reconstruction algorithms [68].

In this chapter, the antenna requirement of this imaging method is discussed. A criteria is proposed for evaluating different antenna structures for synthetic 3D microwave tomography. Finally an efficient antenna structure is proposed for this imaging technique and its performance is evaluated in a simulated imaging scenario.

5.1 Antenna requirement for synthetic 3D microwave tomography

In the synthetic microwave tomography approach, 3D scanning of the IO is achieved using successive 2D scanning at several vertical planes (Fig. 5.1). In the numerical forward solver of the synthetic 3D microwave tomography algo-

rithms, the antenna element should be possible to be efficiently represented as a point-source approximation [68] and [54]. In this approach some approximations have to be accepted, the most important of which are the assumption of the radiated fields to be confined to TM mode and the tissue structure to approximately conform to the cylindrical shape (no sharp deviation in dielectric properties along the cylindrical axis). The more these assumptions match to reality, the more successful the imaging will be. However, in most of the cases some artifact level and clutter have to be tolerated in this imaging technique.
In this imaging procedure antenna elements acting as transmitters and receivers are again among the most important parts of the system directly influencing the efficiency of the imaging. The required specification of an efficient antenna element to be used in practical imaging systems based on synthetic 3D tomography are as follows:

1. High fractional bandwidth to ensure sufficient penetration and good resolution (at frequencies around 3 GHz the inverse problem becomes more ill-posed and therefore more difficult to solve),
2. In synthetic 3D microwave tomography, the antenna should be possible to be efficiently modeled as a point-source scatterer in the numerical 2D forward solver,
3. Possibility of placing a lot of antenna elements around the IO to ensure enough sampling of the scattered electric field and to minimize the clutter and interference in the final reconstructed image,
4. Directional radiation to reduce the interference and to efficiently couple microwave energy into IO is desired.

The goal of this section is to propose a criterion for the evaluation of the performance of antenna elements to be used in synthetic 3D microwave tomography imaging systems. In the previous chapter, through imaging an MRI-derived numerically realistic 2D head model, it was shown that microwave tomography is

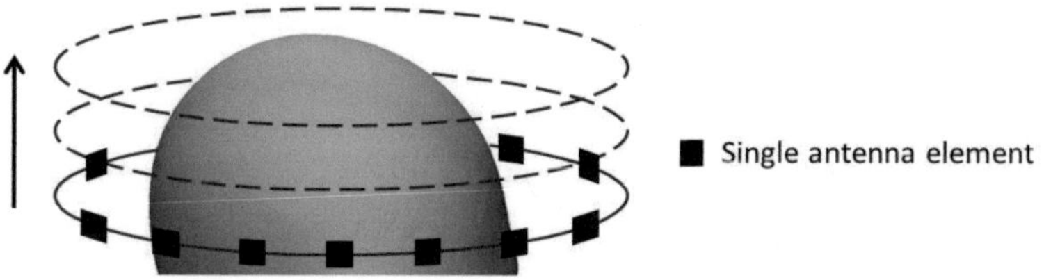

Fig. 5.1: Antenna array surrounding an imaging object in synthetic 3D microwave tomography; successive 2D illumination of IO in several vertical layers.

one promising technique for looking inside the head. Here we are aiming at proposing of an efficient antenna element to be used in practical imaging systems based on synthetic 3D microwave tomography for head imaging as an example application.

In the following sections, first a criterion is proposed for the evaluation of any antenna structure for synthetic 3D microwave tomography. Afterwards the performance of two antenna structures namely the modified Bowtie antenna of the previous section and a Vivaldi antenna are evaluated and compared regarding the proposed criteria for the target application of head imaging. The validity of the proposed criteria is examined by comparing the imaging results of a simulation scenario using two antenna arrays.

5.2 Criteria for the evaluation of antenna elements in synthetic 3D microwave tomography

In synthetic 3D microwave tomography, successive imaging is performed in several vertical layers. The received signals in each layer are processed using 2D image reconstruction algorithms. By combining the results at the end, a 3D image of the object is formed synthetically. Image reconstruction algorithms are

complex nonlinear iterative optimization algorithms. They begin with an approximated 2D numerical model of the imaging setup in each single layer.
To comment on the efficiency of an antenna structure for this imaging procedure, it is necessary to develop a criterion to evaluate the performance of the antenna in the image reconstruction algorithms; i.e. it is necessary to estimate the modeling error as a result of the point-source approximation in the numerical forward solver of the reconstruction algorithm.
In this section the following procedure is proposed for the evaluation of any antenna structure for synthetic 3D microwave tomography:

1. The first evaluation step is to design an imaging setup with actual antennas and either perform a measurement or simulate the setup in a commercial software. In this research, an array of antennas surrounding an imaging tank is simulated in CST microwave studio. The antennas are arranged in the form of a square ring (2D array) (Fig. 5.2).

2. Two 3D simulations are performed with one antenna as the transmitter and all the other antennas in the array as receivers. Assuming N antennas surrounding the tank, N-1 scattering parameters are recorded (S21's). The two simulations are the empty-tank simulation (Fig. 5.2(a)) and the simulation with an imaging object inside the tank (Fig. 5.2(b)).

3. The obtained scattered fields must then be calibrated. There are two main purposes of performing calibration. The first purpose is to convert the measured (or simulated) scattering parameters (S21's) into E field values to be later used in inversion algorithms (the network analyzer measures only the scattering parameters and they have to be converted to E field data). The second very important purpose of calibration is to eliminate or compensate as many measurement errors as possible.

The simulation results are calibrated according to the incident calibration technique [53]; i.e. for each receive antenna a calibrated complex quantity is calculated according to:

$$Sinc, calib = \frac{S_{21,Object} - S_{21,empty}}{S_{21,empty}} \tag{5.1}$$

It has to be noted that every inversion algorithm requires scattered field measurements. However, any physical system is only capable of measuring the total electric field. As a result, first a raw measurement has to be performed to collect the electric field without any scatterer present (the so-called incident electric field). The incident fields are then subtracted from all the subsequent signals to produce the scattered field data (Fig. 5.3).

After the calibration, all the measurement errors that are constant in the two measurements (empty measurement and measurement with object) will be in principle eliminated. Examples of such errors are cable losses and phase shifts as a result of different cable lengths. However, other source of errors that vary between the two measurements will not be totally removed; e.g. the coupling between the adjacent antenna elements are influenced by the presence of the imaging objects and therefore will not be totally removed. Such uncompensated errors will deteriorate the inversion efficiency and will show up as clutter in the final reconstructed images.

4. The imaging setup of CST is afterwards numerically modeled in a forward solver. In this research the FDTD-based solver MEEP is used [52]. In the 2D numerical model of MEEP, actual antennas are replaced by ideal point sources (Fig. 5.4).

5. Two MEEP simulations are performed with and without the IO inside the tank (Fig. 5.4 (a) and (b)). After each simulation, N-1 electric fields are recorded at the position of receive point sources. The electric fields are afterwards calibrated according to:

$$Einc,calib = \frac{E_{object} - E_{empty}}{E_{empty}} \tag{5.2}$$

6. For the evaluation of the performance of the antenna, the modeling error is estimated as the mean square error (MSE) between the calibrated S parameters of CST with actual antennas and the calibrated electric field of MEEP (equations (5.1) and (5.2)) calculated using point-source approximation.

5.3 Comparison of two antenna structures for application in synthetic 3D microwave tomography

In order to propose an efficient antenna structure for application in synthetic 3D microwave tomography, we examine and compare the performance of two antenna elements namely the previously proposed modified Bowtie antenna and a Vivaldi antenna optimized for biomedical imaging.

5.3.1 Modified Bowtie antenna

The modified Bowtie antenna was initially designed and optimized for full wave 3D microwave tomography in the previous chapter (Fig. 5.5). With the radiation of the antenna being independent of its feeding network, the antenna model in the 3D numerical forward solver could be simplified to the radiative (Bowtie) element and it was shown that there is no need to include the feeding of the antenna in the numerical model.

5.3.2 Vivaldi antenna

In [54] and [17], a Vivaldi antenna was exploited in air-based microwave tomography imaging systems. In this research a Vivaldi structure is optimized for

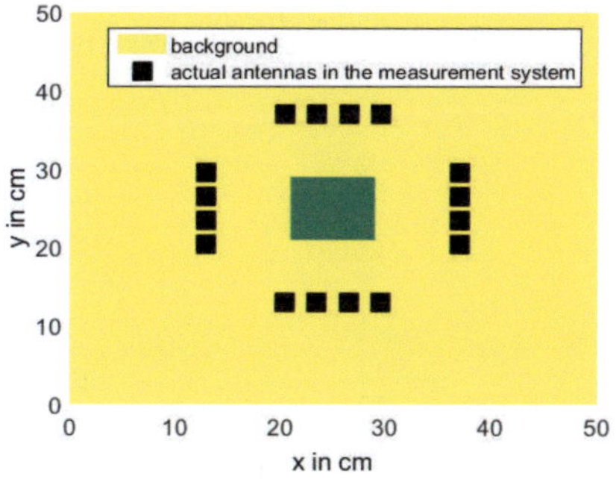

(a)

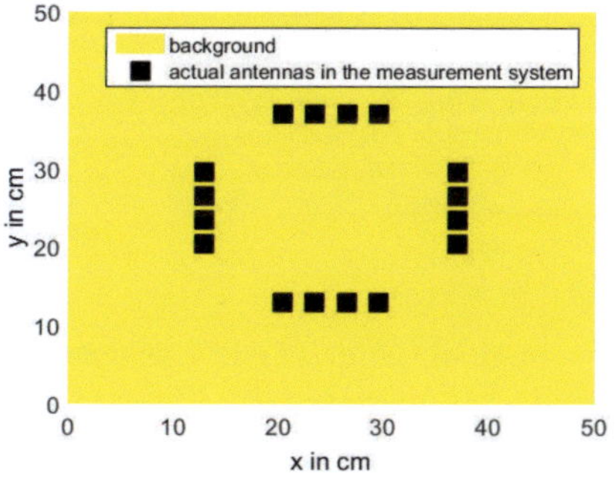

(b)

Fig. 5.2: A view of the 3D CST imaging setup consisting of an array of actual antennas around an imaging tank; (a) imaging object inside the tank (b) empty tank.

medical imaging application and its performance is evaluated for application in synthetic 3D microwave tomography. For the optimum transfer of the input signal to the object the Vivaldi antenna was optimized with the front part of the antenna inside the matching medium (ethanol-water solution) and the rear part of the antenna in air (Fig. 5.6). The final antenna was 3 cm inside a matching medium of relative permittivity of 45 and conductivity of 0.5 S/m (at 1 GHz).

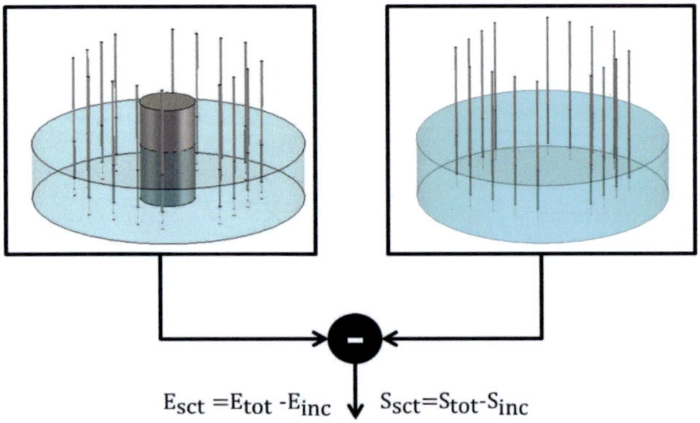

Fig. 5.3: Two successive simulations (measurements) are performed (with object and without object) to determine the scattered field.

The optimum frequency range of 0.5 to 2 GHz was considered in the design and optimization of the antenna. The substrate was Rogers 4003 (relative permittivity of 3.55, loss tangent 0.0027 and thickness of 1.53 mm) and the dimension of the antenna was 73 mm x 50 mm. The detailed structure of the antenna and some important dimension are displayed and listed in Fig. 5.6 and Table 5.1.

Tabelle 5.1: Detailed dimension of the Vivaldi antenna

L	W	R	k	d	t
73 mm	50 mm	20 mm	19 mm	3.5 mm	0.37 mm

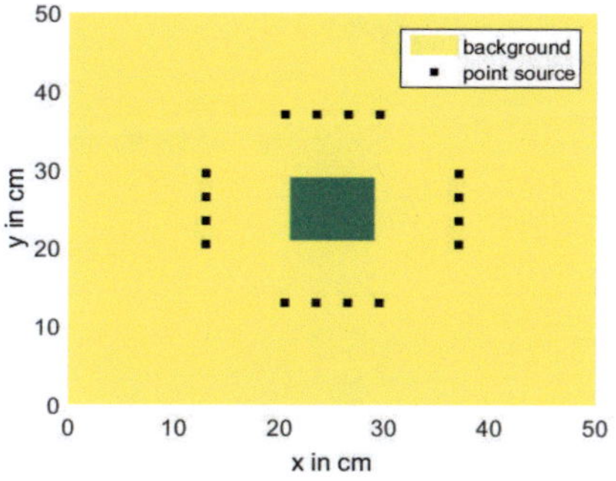

(a)

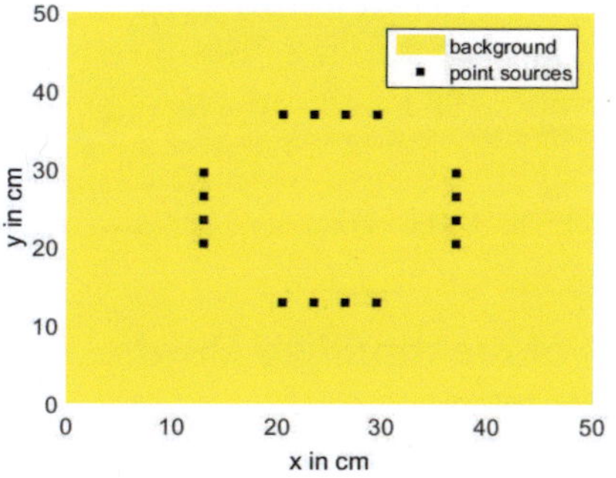

(b)

Fig. 5.4: 2D numerical model of the imaging system consisting of an array of point-source antennas around an imaging tank (a) imaging object inside the tank (b) empty tank.

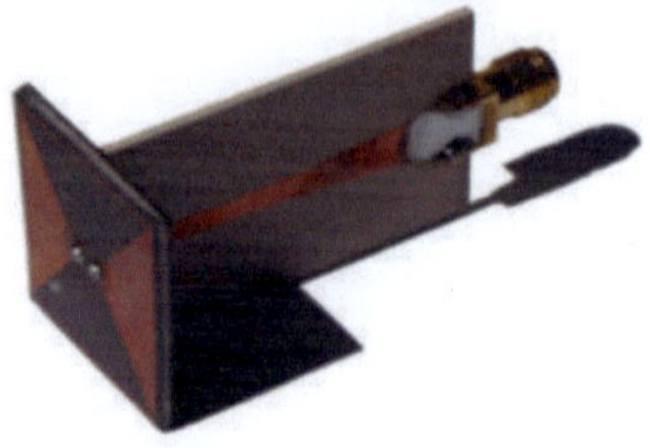

Fig. 5.5: The modified Bowtie antenna proposed for full-wave 3D microwave tomography in Chapter 4.

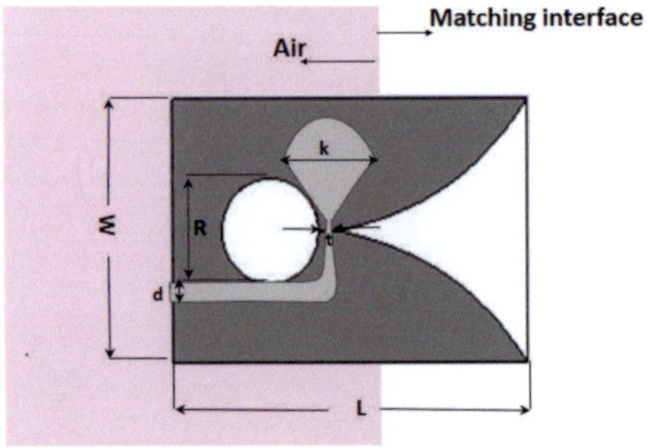

Fig. 5.6: The detailed structure of the Vivaldi antenna.

5.3.3 Comparison of the modified Bowtie and Vivaldi antennas

Reflection coefficient

The simulated reflection coefficients of the two antennas are compared in Fig. 5.7. From the comparison of the two S11 curves, it turns out that the Bowtie antenna exhibits a better matching through the whole frequency range up to 2GHz. Table 5.2 presents a review of some specifications of the two antennas.

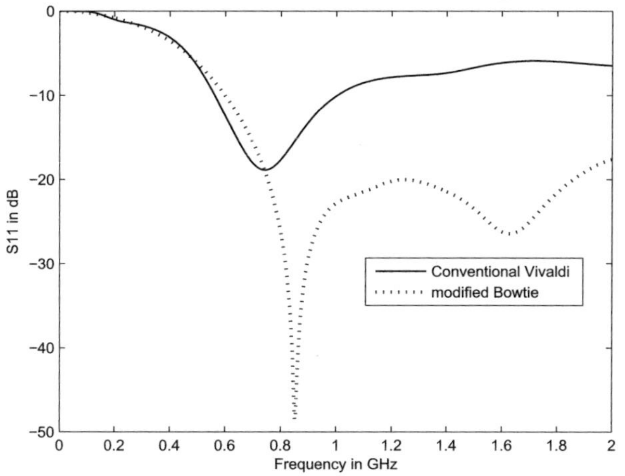

Fig. 5.7: The simulated reflection coefficient of the Bowtie and Vivaldi antennas.

Tabelle 5.2: Comparison of the Bowtie and Vivaldi antennas - I

	Bowtie	Conventional Vivaldi
Operational bandwidth	0.6-2 GHz	0.5-1.5 GHz
Dimension in mm	22 x 22	73 x 50

Modeling error as a result of point source approximation in the 2D numerical solver

The two antenna structures are further compared regarding their performance in synthetic 3D microwave tomography using the criteria proposed previously in this chapter.

Two separate imaging setups are built in CST microwave studio (Fig. 5.8 and Fig. 5.9). Both CST simulations involve an imaging tank (width 24 cm; height 10 cm) filled with matching liquid having a relative permittivity of 45 and conductivity of 0.5 S/m at 1 GHz. In two different simulations, 16 antennas are inserted into the walls of this tank with the distance between adjacent antennas equal to 3 cm. One of the CST imaging setups was a 2D antenna array composed of 16 Bowtie elements (Fig. 5.8) whereas the second imaging setup was that of 16 Vivaldi antennas inserted into the walls of the same tank (Fig. 5.9). For each CST imaging setup the following two simulations were performed:

1. Empty tank simulation: In this simulation there is no object inside the tank (except for the interface liquid (Fig. 5.8 (a) and (b) and Fig. 5.9 (a) and (b))). With the first antenna as the transmitter, 15 S-parameters are recorded (S21-empty) by the other antennas (CST spatial resolution $\frac{\lambda}{30}$).

2. Imaging object inside the tank: In this simulation, a square cylinder of size 8 cm (permittivity 60 and conductivity 1 S/m) is placed in the middle of the tank with the interface liquid surrounding it (Fig. 5.8 (c) and (d)). Once again, with the first antenna as the transmitter, 15 scattered signals are recorded by the receive antennas (S21-Object) in both imaging setups.

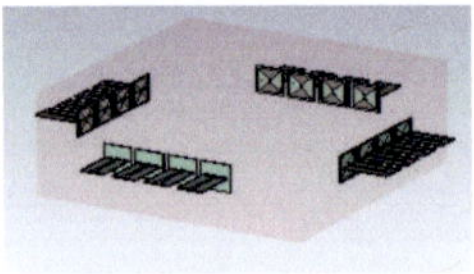

(a) Empty chamber (view1)

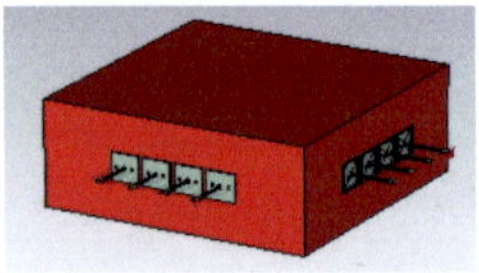

(b) Empty chamber (view2)

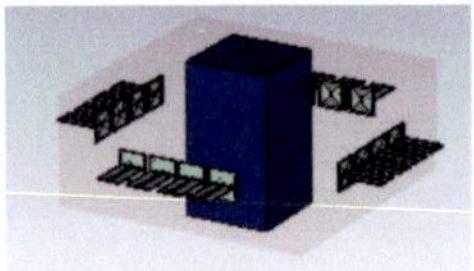

(c) Target inside (view1)

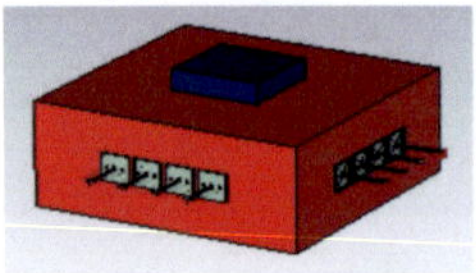

(d) Target inside (view2)

Fig. 5.8: CST simulation model: 16 Bowtie antennas on the wall of an imaging tank filled with matching interface; (a) and (b) empty chamber, (c) and (d) square cylinder in the middle of the chamber.

The recorded signals are calibrated using incident calibration technique; i.e. for each receive antenna a calibrated complex quantity is calculated according to 5.1. After obtaining the calibrated signals corresponding to the Bowtie and Vi-

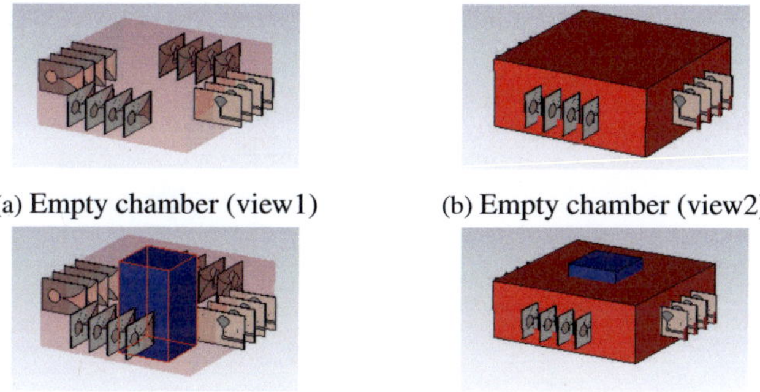

(a) Empty chamber (view1) (b) Empty chamber (view2)

(c) Target inside (view1) (d) Target inside (view2)

Fig. 5.9: CST simulation model: 16 Vivaldi antennas partly inside a matching interface; (a) and (b) empty chamber, (c) and (d) square cylinder in the middle of the chamber.

valdi antenna arrays in CST, the two imaging setups are modeled in the numerical MEEP solver. A 2D numerical model representing both of the Bowtie and Vivaldi imaging setups is simulated as shown in Fig. 5.10. In the MEEP model, the actual Bowtie and Vivaldi antennas are replaced by 16 ideal point source elements.

Following a similar procedure as in CST, two 2D simulations were performed in MEEP; i.e. empty-tank simulation and simulation with the square object. The scattered electric fields were estimated at the position of the point-source receivers and the results were calibrated according to the equation 5.2.

In Fig. 5.11 and 5.12, the amplitude and phase of the calibrated signals obtained from the actual antennas in CST and the corresponding point source approximations in MEEP are compared together at four frequencies from 0.5 to 2 GHz. As observed in the figures, for the Bowtie array the deviation of the calibrated amplitude and phase from the calibrated MEEP results for some receive antennas is quite high up to 1.5 GHz (especially higher than the corresponding values of the Vivaldi antennas). Above 1.5 GHz, however, the MSE error of Bowtie antenna is lower. The mean square error (MSE) between the signals obtained by the antennas and the MEEP point sources are reported in Table. 5.3.

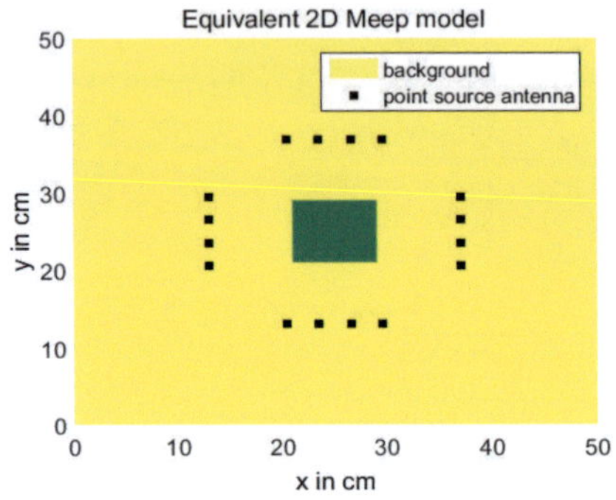

Fig. 5.10: The numerical model of the two CST simulation setups (Bowtie array and Vivaldi array) in MEEP.

Tabelle 5.3: Comparison of the three antennas - II

	modified Bowtie	Conventional Vivaldi
2D modeling error @ 0.5 GHz	15.546%	6.975%
2D modeling error @ 1 GHz	10.575%	6.599%
2D modeling error @ 1.5 GHz	6.601%	6.736%
2D modeling error @ 2 GHz	1.111%	9.725%

Therefore, although the Bowtie antenna has a lower reflection coefficient up to 2 GHz relative to the Vivaldi antenna, the proposed criteria predicts lower imaging efficiency using the Bowtie array at some frequencies. Later in this chapter, the validity of the proposed criteria will be examined in a simulated imaging scenario.

In the following, the two antenna structures are further compared using a second criterion to find out which antenna directs more power into the IO and therefore is expected to yield a higher signal to noise ratio in the imaging system.

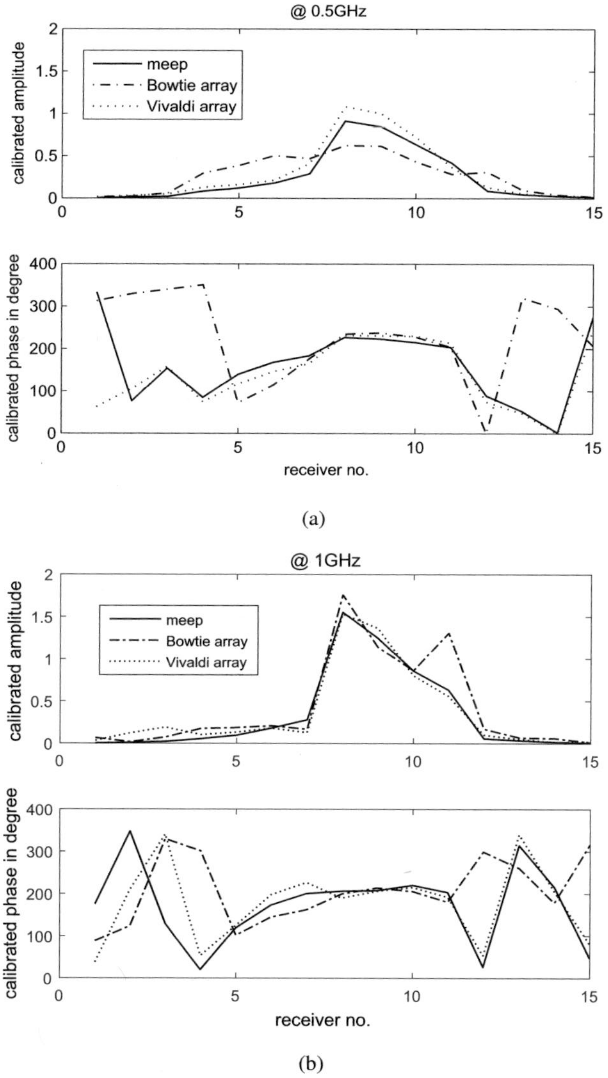

Fig. 5.11: The comparison of the calibrated received signals of CST and MEEP. (a) F= 0.5 GHz; (b) F= 1 GHz.

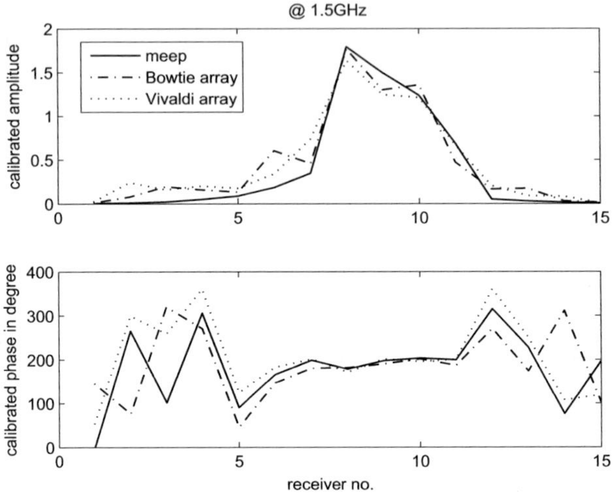

(a)

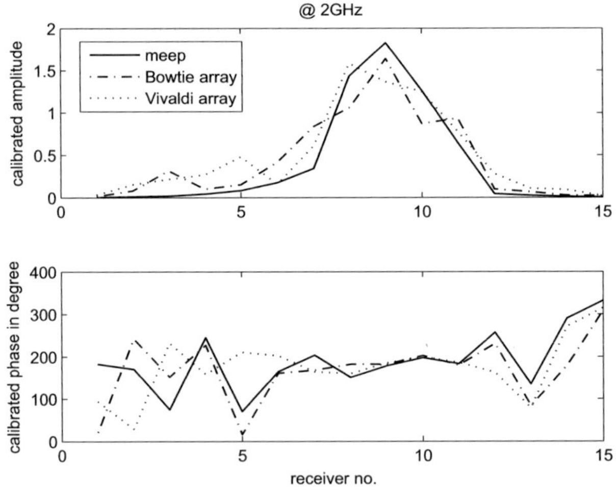

(b)

Fig. 5.12: The comparison of the calibrated received signals of CST and MEEP. (a) F= 1.5 GHz; (b) F= 2 GHz.

Coupled power into an imaging object

To compare the efficiency of the modified Bowtie and conventional Vivaldi antennas in coupling microwave power into an IO, the same criterion as in chapter 4 is used in that the two antennas are placed at the same distance (60 mm) to a multilayer head model (biggest dimension 140 mm) and the coupled power to the head model is estimated via simulations in CST microwave studio.
The absolute value of the coupled power into the head model with the Vivaldi antenna at the distance of 40 mm to the model is represented in Fig. 5.13 at four different frequencies. The results can be compared to the corresponding power values of the Bowtie antenna in the previous chapter. For a more quantitative comparison, the absolute values of the total power (in dB) at a reference line in the middle of the head model are extracted and compared in Fig. 5.14 at four frequencies. It is observed in the figure that the Vivaldi antenna succeeds in coupling more power into the head model in the whole frequency range of 0.5 to 2 GHz.
The Vivaldi antenna is afterwards fabricated on Rogers 4003 substrate (permittivity of 3.55, loss tangent 0.0027 and thickness of 1.53 mm) (see Fig. 5.15). The reflection coefficient of the fabricated antenna is then measured in a matching liquid of ethanol-water solution. 3 cm of antenna's radiating part is inserted into the liquid (Fig. 5.16 (a)) while the rest of the antenna is in air. In Fig. 5.16 (b) the simulated S11 is compared to the corresponding measured values.
It can be concluded that the Vivaldi antenna outperforms the Bowtie antenna considering the lower modeling error in the image reconstruction algorithms. The Vivaldi antenna also represents a superior performance regarding the transfer of the microwave power to an IO (example multilayer head model). It was shown that the better matching of the Bowtie antenna in this imaging procedure doesn't lead to a necessarily better performance. Additionally, the longitudinal structure of the Vivaldi antenna allows placing more antenna elements around an IO and therefore makes efficient sampling of the scattered signals possible. The-

refore, the Vivaldi antenna is introduced as an efficient structure for synthetic microwave tomography imaging systems. In the following section, the imaging capabilities of the two antenna structures will be further examined and compared in a simulation scenario for head imaging.

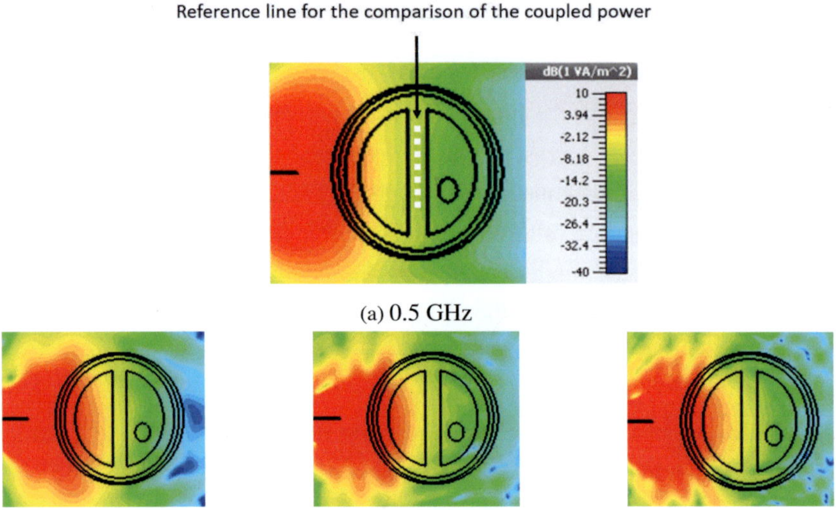

(a) 0.5 GHz

(b) 1 GHz

(c) 1.5 GHz

(d) 2 GHz

Fig. 5.13: The Vivaldi antenna illuminating the multilayer head model in CST microwave studio. Absolute E-field at (a) 0.5 GHz, (b)1GHz, (c) 1.5 GHz and (d) 2 GHz.

5.4 Microwave tomography imaging system - detection of hemorrhagic stroke

In the previous sections, a criterion was proposed to compare the performance of the modified Bowtie antenna to the Vivaldi antenna for application in synthetic 3D microwave tomography. By estimating the modeling error corresponding to both antenna arrays, it turned out that the Vivaldi antenna outperforms the Bow-tie antenna in spite of the better matching of the Bowtie in the whole frequency

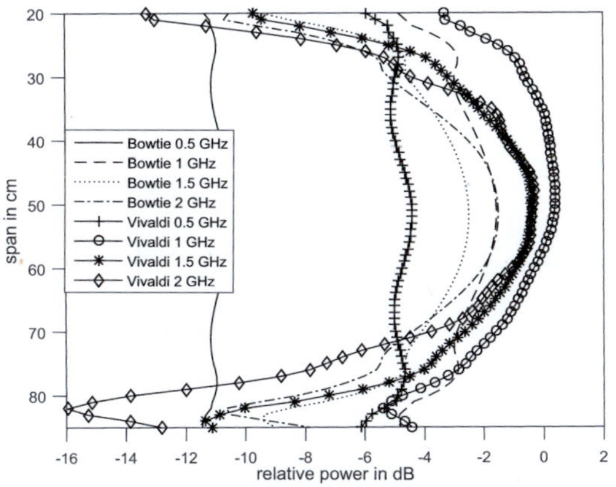

Fig. 5.14: Coupled power to the head model at a reference line in the middle of the head (see Fig. 5.13 (a))- comparison of Vivaldi to Bowtie antenna

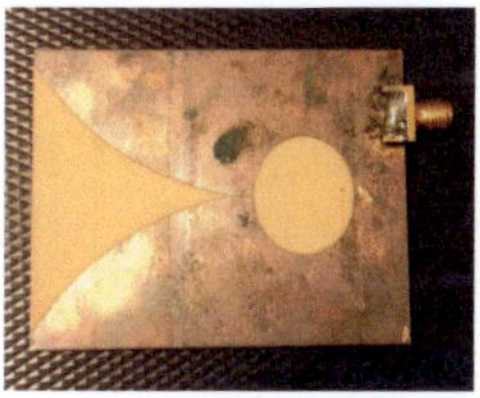

(a) Radiative side

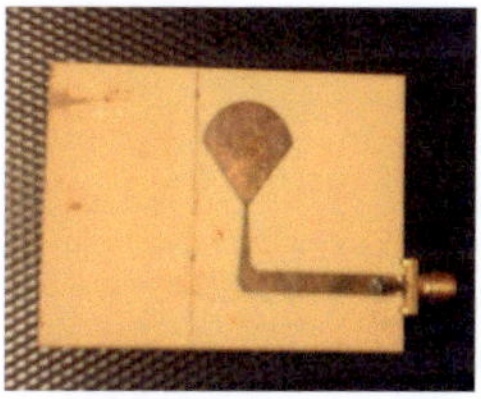

(b) Feeding network

Fig. 5.15: The fabricated Vivaldi antenna.

range of interest. In this section, the goal is to prove the validity of the proposed criteria for the evaluation of the performance of antennas.

For this purpose, two imaging scenarios are simulated in CST microwave studio. The performance of the Bowtie and Vivaldi antenna arrays are evaluated regarding the detection of a hemorrhagic stroke inside the white matter of a multilayer head model. The multilayer head model with dispersive layers is the one used before for the evaluation of the antennas in chapter 4 (see Fig. 5.17). The head model is placed inside an imaging tank (width 24 cm, height 100 cm) filled with

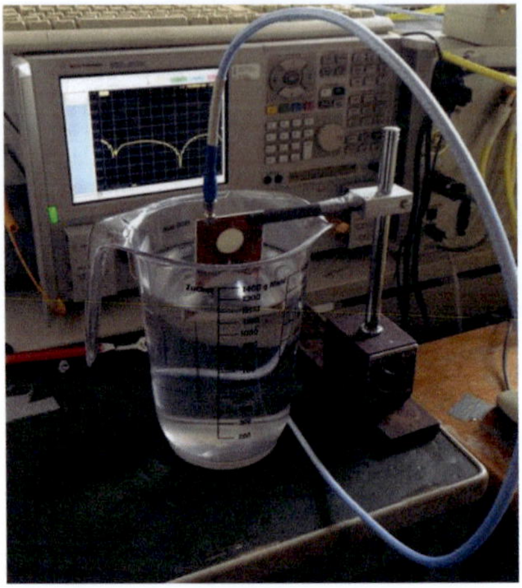

(a) Measurement setup

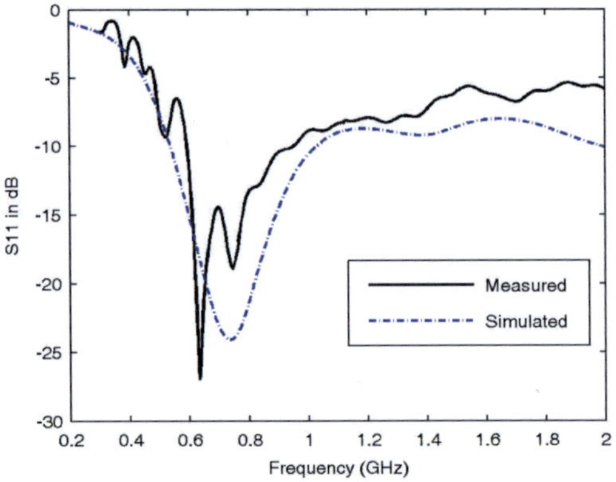

(b) Simulated and measured reflection coefficients

Fig. 5.16: Reflection coefficient of the Vivaldi antenna: (a) measurement setup, (b) the comparison of the simulated and measured values.

Tabelle 5.4: Dielectric characteristics of CST head phantom at 1 GHz

	skin	skull	gray matter	white matter	stroke
Permittivty	45.71	12.36	52.28	38.58	61
Conductivity (S / m)	0.88	0.155	0.98	0.62	2

a matching interface of relative permittivity 45 and conductivity of 0.5 S/m at 1 GHz. In two separate imaging projects 16 antennas are inserted into the walls of the tank; i.e. 16 Bowtie antennas in the first project (Fig. 5.18(a)) and 16 Vivaldi antennas in the second project (Fig. 5.18(b)). The following simulations are performed in CST microwave studio (for both imaging setups):

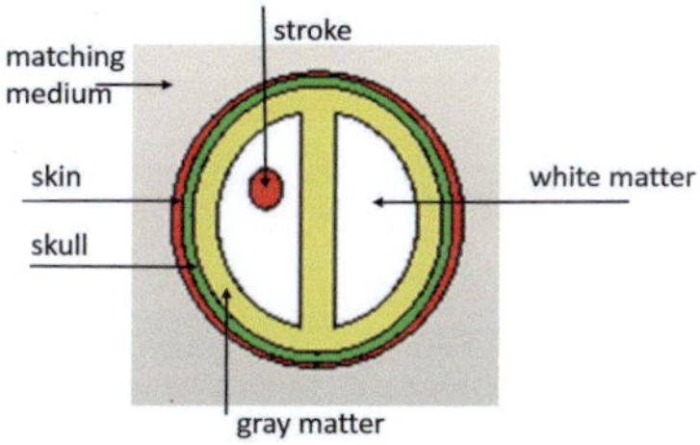

Fig. 5.17: The multilayer head model simulated in CST. The dielectric properties of the layers are listed in Table 5.4

5.4.1 Empty tank simulation

In this simulation with no object inside the tank (except for the interface liquid (Fig. 5.18)) following a multistatic scenario, 240 S- parameters were recorded (S21-empty).

5.4.2 Head phantom inside the tank

The multilayer head model is afterwards simulated inside the tank with the interface medium surrounding it (Fig. 5.19 (a) and (b)). Once again, following a multistatic scenario 240 scattered signals were recorded (S21-head). The recorded signals are then calibrated using incident calibration technique (equation 5.1). The calibrated signals are used as the input to the iterative nonlinear reconstruction unit based on Gauss-Newton optimization.

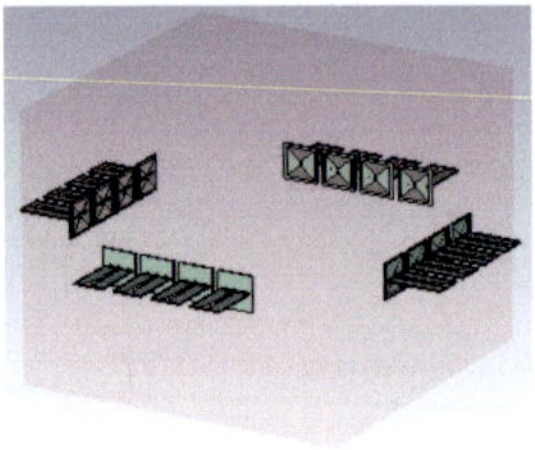

(a) Bowtie array

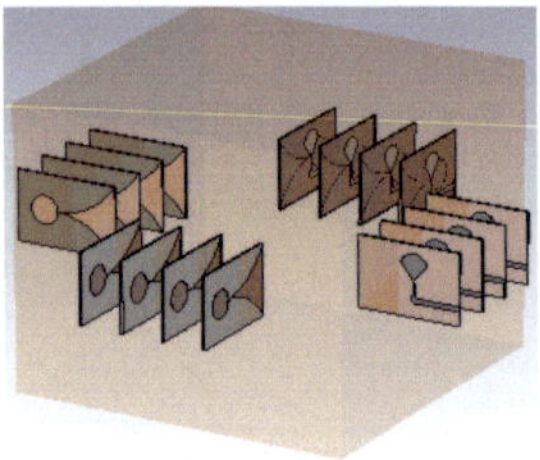

(b) Vivaldi array

Fig. 5.18: The Vivaldi array and Bowtie array surrounding the tank filled with matching liquid in CST Microwave Studio.

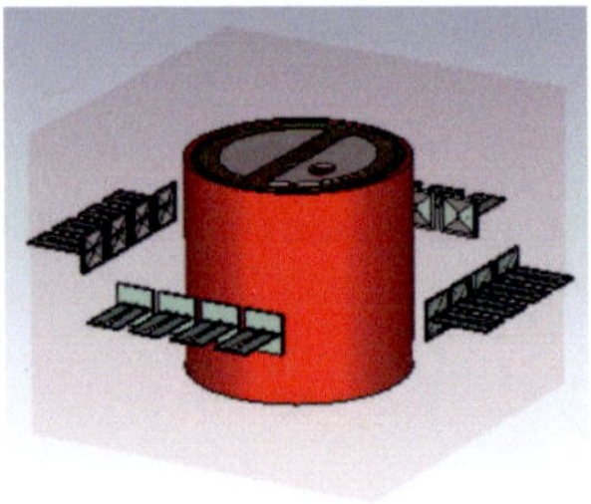

(a) Bowtie array

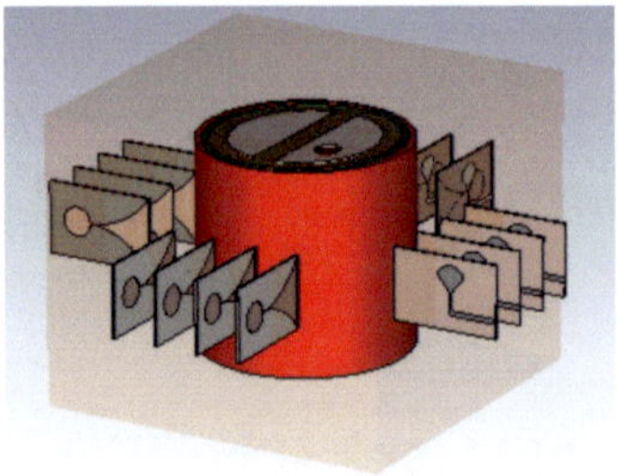

(b) Vivaldi array

Fig. 5.19: The Vivaldi array and Bowtie array surrounding the multilayer head model in CST Microwave Studio.

The image reconstruction procedure used in this chapter is the iterative nonlinear Gauss-Newton algorithm exploited in Chapter 3. No priori information about the head phantom (shape of the layers or the dielectric properties of single tissues) is assumed. In the first iteration (initial guess) all the mesh cells (90×90 mesh cells) are assumed to have the dielectric properties of the matching medium

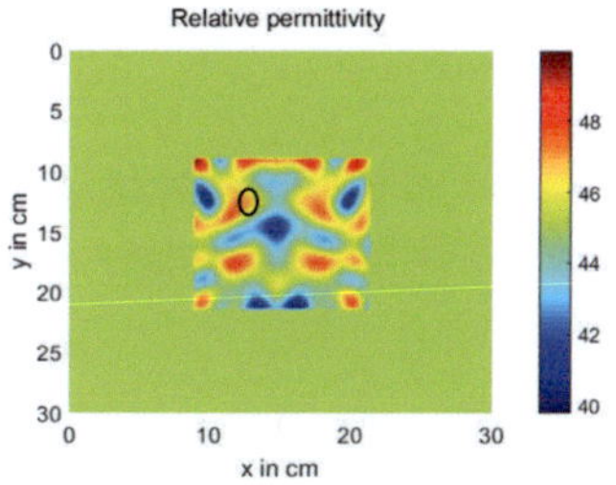

(a) relative permittivity- 1st iteration

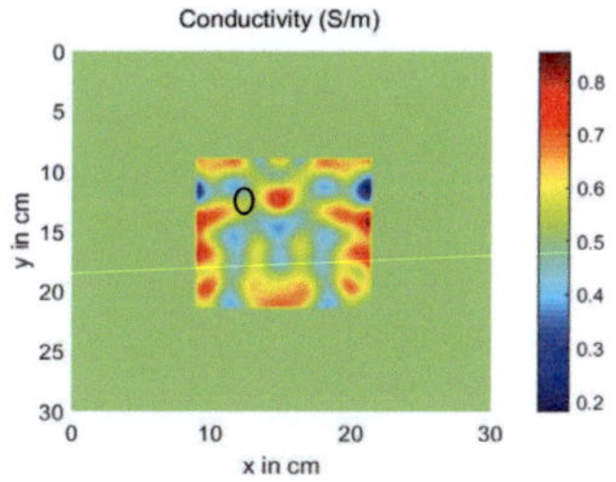

(b) conductivity (S/m)- 1st iteration

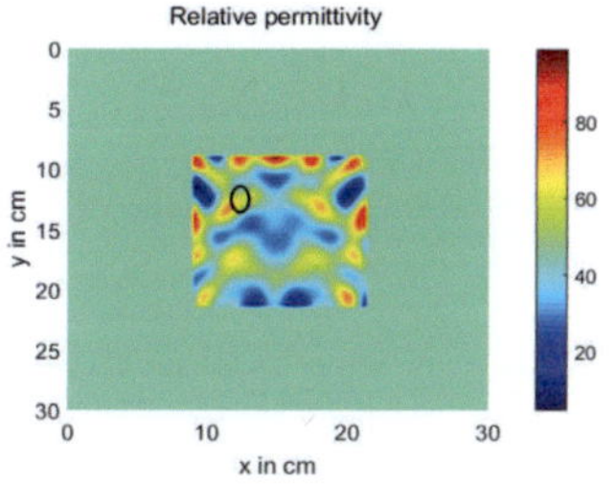

(c) relative permittivity- 24th iteration

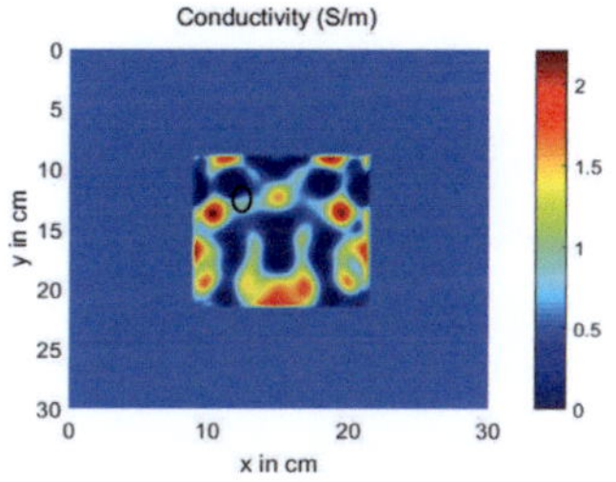

(d) conductivity (S/m)- 24th iteration

Fig. 5.20: The imaging results using Bowtie array at 1GHz. (a) and (b) results after the first iteration. (c) and (d) final results (the black circle shows the position of the stroke in the original simulated model).

(blind reconstruction). The imaging is performed at the single frequency of 1 GHz and the Bowtie and Vivaldi antennas are represented by 16 point-sources in the forward solver MEEP. Since the imaging setups are identical except for the structure of the antennas, the same numerical model is used for the image reconstruction of both antenna arrays (Fig. 5.10).

Figs. 5.20 (a) and (b) and 5.21 (a) and (b) show the reconstructed images of both the Bowtie and Vivaldi arrays right after the first iteration. By comparing the reconstructed image of the Vivaldi array to the Bowtie array, it is clearly observed that the general shape of the head model and even the stroke area inside the white matter are clearly visible in case of the Vivaldi array right after the first iteration. The imaging result corresponding to the Bowtie array presents little information about the simulated head model. It even seems as if the stroke area has not yet been sensed by the Bowtie antennas although the reconstructed image is symmetrical.

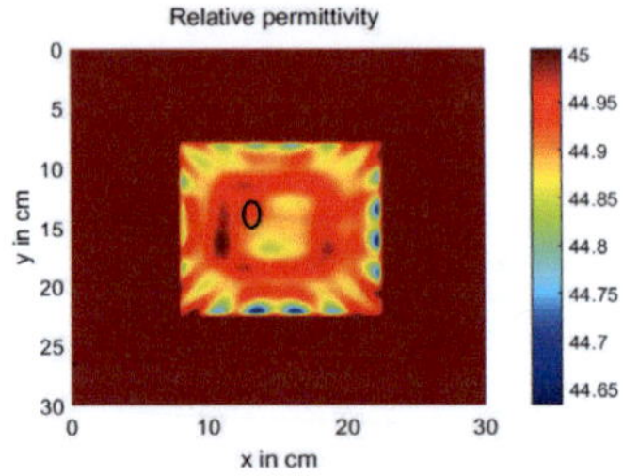

(a) relative permittivity- 1st iteration

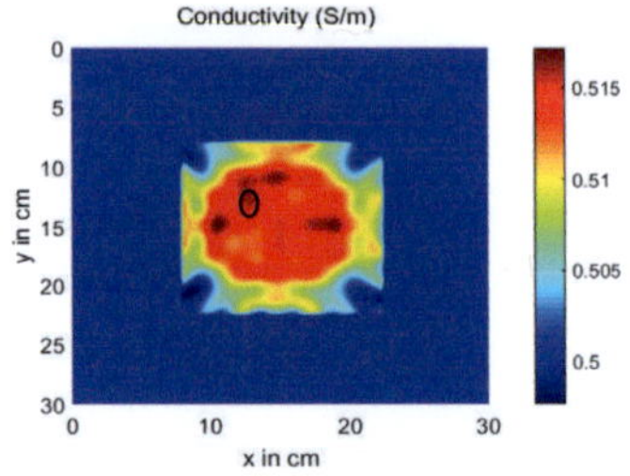

(b) conductivity (S/m)- 1st iteration

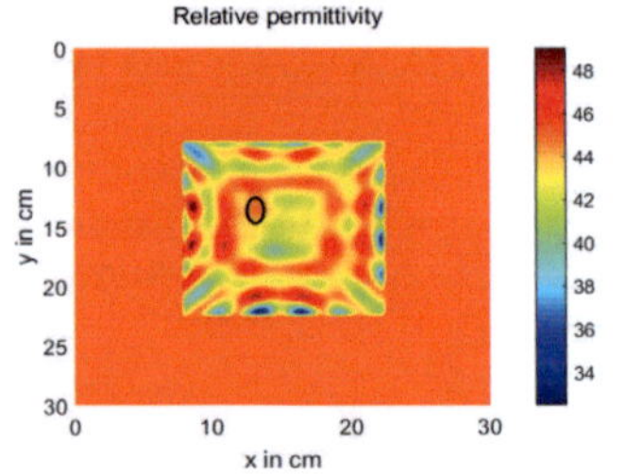

(c) relative permittivity- 24th iteration

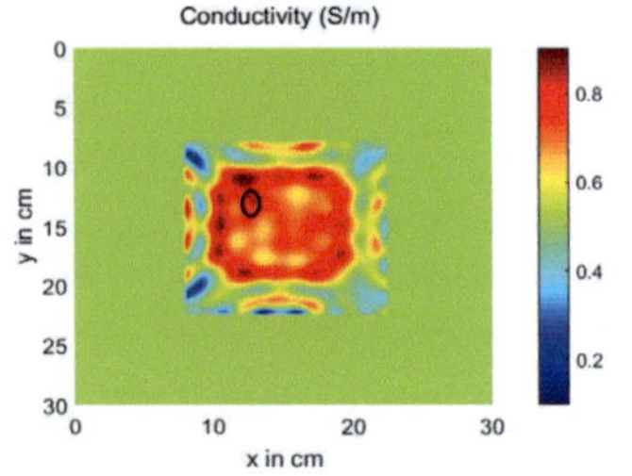

(d) conductivity (S/m)- 24th iteration

Fig. 5.21: The imaging results using Vivaldi array at 1GHz. (a) and (b) results after the first iteration. (c) and (d) final results (the black circle shows the position of the stroke in the original simulated model).

The quantitative imaging results after 24 iterations are presented in Figs . 5.20 (c) and (d) and 5.21 (c) and (d). As can be seen, in case of the Vivaldi array even with a mono-frequency reconstruction approach, the stroke area is clearly reconstructed and detected in both permittivity and conductivity profiles although the quantitative values do not exactly converge to the actual ones. As shown in [58] and [5], multiple-frequency approach can be applied to improve the results quantitatively and qualitatively. The wide bandwidth of the antennas supports the application of this technique. This subject, however, was not within the focus of this work.

In conclusion, a Vivaldi antenna was proposed for application in synthetic 3D microwave tomography and its performance was compared to the modified Bow-tie antenna of chapter 4. The superior performance of the Vivaldi antenna predicted by the modeling error criteria was confirmed by the imaging results of the simulated multilayer head model. The use of the proposed criteria brings furthermore the following additional advantages for the optimization of the imaging procedure:

1. The dimension of the imaging tank and the antenna array configuration affect the imaging results in synthetic 3D microwave tomography. The proposed criterion assists in pre-optimization of the tank and the placement of the antennas in a way to minimize the modeling error between the actual imaging system and the numerical model representing the system in the numerical forward solver of the image reconstruction unit.

2. The criterion further assists in the choice of the optimum frequency of operation. Above all, the frequencies at which a high modeling error is predicted by the criteria, should be avoided in the imaging procedure. This is because it was shown in this chapter that a high modeling error leads to poor imaging results.

3. The criterion also helps comparing the performance of different antenna structures without performing actual imaging. This was confirmed in this chapter by the comparison of the modeling error corresponding to the Bowtie antenna and the Vivaldi antenna.

It has to be mentioned that the Vivaldi antenna can in principle be used for full-wave 3D microwave tomography as well. Compared to the modified Bowtie antenna recommended in chapter 4, the longitudinal structure of the antenna allows placing more elements around the IO (off-set 3D locations). However, since in 3D microwave tomography the antenna array needs to be numerically modeled in the reconstruction algorithms, the larger dimension of the Vivaldi antenna (73 mm) exposes more computational load to the imaging procedure than the Bowtie antenna (22 mm).

6 Efficient antenna for Radar beamforming

As discussed in the first Chapter, for imaging applications with a high contrast between the target and the neighboring tissues (e.g. tumor detection in breast), it is possible to use qualitative imaging techniques and therefore to avoid the otherwise computationally extensive quantitative approaches (microwave tomography). The imaging setup includes an array of antennas surrounding an IO and illuminating it with broadband signals in either a monostatic or multistatic approach (Fig. 6.1). The different imaging algorithms in this technique compete in generating a clutter-free energy map of the target showing the position of strong scatterers inside it ([73], [31], [10], [14], [21], [51], [4], [28]).

The final goal of microwave imaging technology is the development of a low-cost and reliable imaging system that can be easily adopted to clinical situations. UWB antennas play an important role in realizing successful and efficient imaging systems. To maximize the number of antennas to receive more information from the scattered signal, the size of antenna should be as small as possible. Planar antennas with quasi constant phase center are the best option for this purpose. The modified Bowtie antenna was initially proposed in chapter 4 as an efficient structure for application in full-wave 3D microwave tomography. The antenna with its planar configuration and its wide bandwidth is an efficient option for conformal imaging array solutions.

In this chapter, first the required specification of UWB antennas for microwave Radar imaging technique are discussed. Afterwards the performance of the Bowtie antenna is evaluated in two implemented imaging systems for the detection of stroke in a human head-mimicking phantom and for breast cancer detection.

For the breast tumor detection, however, the antenna is re-optimized to better match the required specification of the application.

6.1 Antenna requirement for microwave Radar imaging

For the successful operation of Radar-based imaging systems that are based on illuminating the target with UWB signals, the antenna under the test should fulfill the following requirements:

1. efficient directional transmission of power into the IO,
2. compact nature for enabling integration of a large number of elements in the antenna array,
3. ability to transmit and receive signals in a broad frequency range, including both low and high frequencies, in order to guarantee high resolution as well as good penetration inside biological tissues

Most of the antennas proposed so far for Radar imaging systems (e.g. [36], [25], [26], [77], [44], [35]), cover the spectrum of nearly 4 to 10 GHz, which corresponds to a fractional bandwidth of 85%. However, to ensure sufficient penetration into the breast tissue (especially into the low-adipose tissues [30]) radiation down to lower frequencies around 1 GHz is favorable. Since the dimension of the antenna is wavelength-dependent, the design of a compact antenna that covers lower frequencies is quite a challenge.

6.2 Miniaturized UWB antenna for breast imaging

In qualitative Radar imaging, it is desired to have a compact UWB antenna element that will efficiently transmit and receive signals with a minimal distortion. The broadband Bowtie antenna with its stable phase center is a very suitable

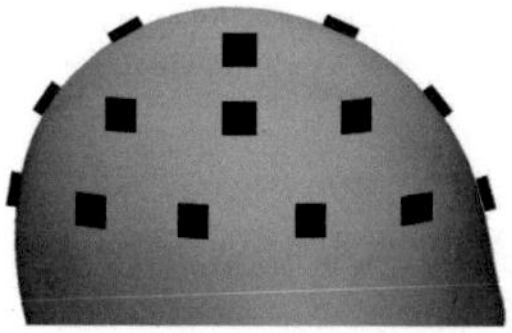

Fig. 6.1: Conformal antenna array surrounding an imaging object in Radar approach.

choice for this approach. The antenna presented in this section is an optimized version of the Bowtie antenna presented in chapter 4 for full-wave 3D microwave tomography. With the two arms of the conventional Bowtie antenna being short-connected (see Fig. 6.2 (a)), the capacitive nature of the antenna is partly compensated and therefore, it is possible to optimize the dimension of the antenna so that it will radiate efficiently in a broadband spectrum. The balun transition of the feeding structure also leads to a symmetrical radiation in the bandwidth of interest.

For breast cancer detection using UWB Radar, the antenna proposed in chapter 4 has been further optimized to cover a wide frequency range starting from around 1 GHz to ensure good penetration into the breast. Therefore the Bowtie was either in direct contact to a breast-mimicking phantom or inside a matching liquid representing an average relative permittivity of $\varepsilon = 20$. The feeding balun must be, however, inside a low-permittivity environment to ensure the directional radiation of the antenna into the phantom or matching liquid.

The structure of the optimized antenna can be seen in Fig. 6.2. The radiating part of the antenna has a compact dimension of 15 mm. The feeding network and the Bowtie are constructed on different substrates. Rogers 5880 with relative permittivity of 2.2 and thickness of 1.57 mm is used for the radiating Bowtie. To ensure reasonable dimension of the feeding network in comparison to the

Bowtie, Rogers 6110 with a relative permittivity of 10.2 and thickness of 1.27 mm is used for the feeding.

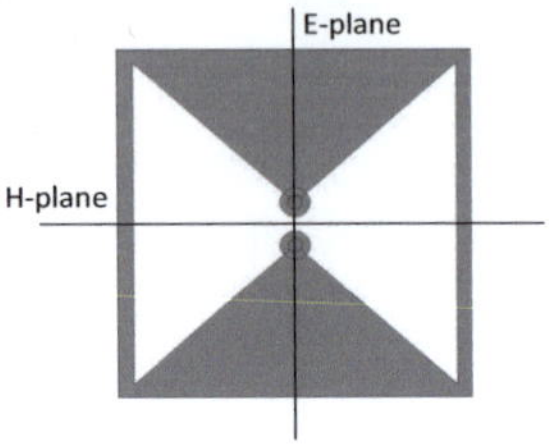

(a)

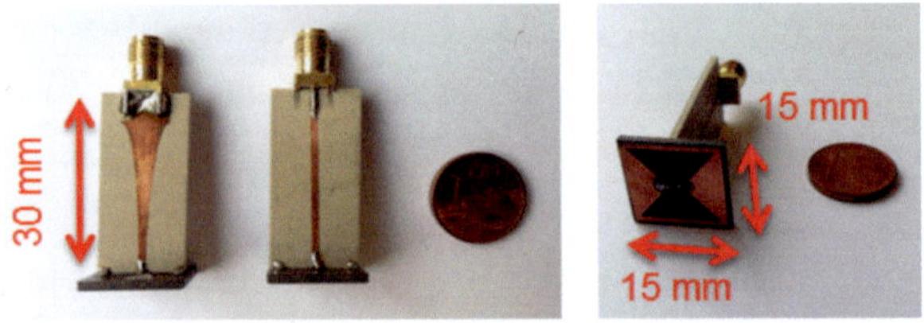

(b)

Fig. 6.2: The modified Bowtie antenna with the inductive strips and the balun feeding; (a) schematic of the antenna, (b) different views of the manufactured antenna.

The reflectivity of the designed antenna is measured with the Bowtie inside a PEG (polyethylene glycol)-water solution having a relative permittivity of 18 at 4 GHz, while the feeding network is kept in air. In Fig. 6.3 the simulated and measured reflection coefficients of the antenna are displayed. It is observed both in simulation and measurement that the reflectivity of the antenna stays below -8 dB in the bandwidth of 1.2 - 7 GHz.

The simulated electric field of the antenna is displayed in Fig. 6.4. As observed in the figures, the electric field begins to radiate into two separate directions starting from 7 GHz (Fig. 6.4 (d)). The radiated field of the antenna is further measured using the near-field imaging system [34] and the measured radiation in E-plane and H-plane are displayed in Fig. 6.5. Since in near-field imaging we are interested in directional antennas, in this case the frequencies higher than 7 GHz

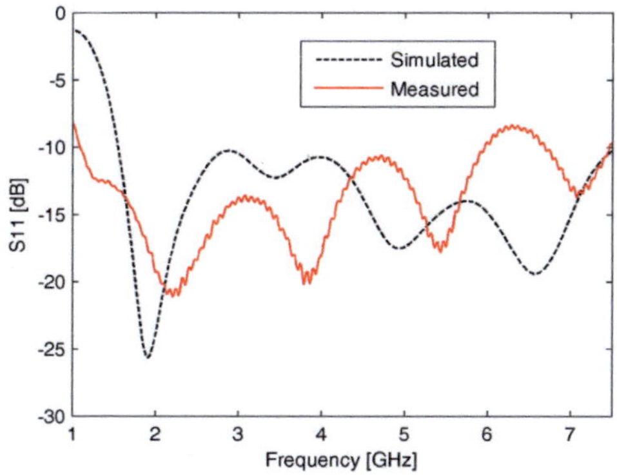

Fig. 6.3: The simulated and measured reflection coefficient of the Bowtie antenna in the PEG solution for breast cancer detection.

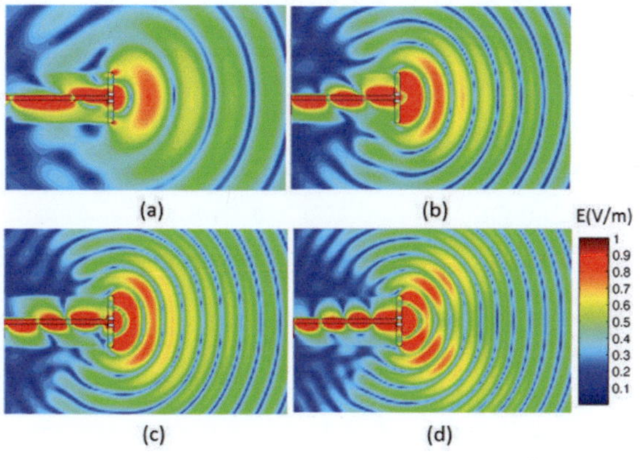

Fig. 6.4: Simulated normalized electric field distribution of the antenna (in the near-field region) with the background permittivity of 20 at (a) 4 GHz, (b) 5 GHz, (c) 6 GHz and (d) 7 GHz.

are not practical. Therefore, the compact Bowtie antenna having a maximum dimension of 15 mm x 15 mm and a bandwidth of 1.2-7 GHz (corresponding to a fractional bandwidth of 141.46%) is in the next chapter used in our near-field imaging system for detection of tumor in synthesized breast phantoms.

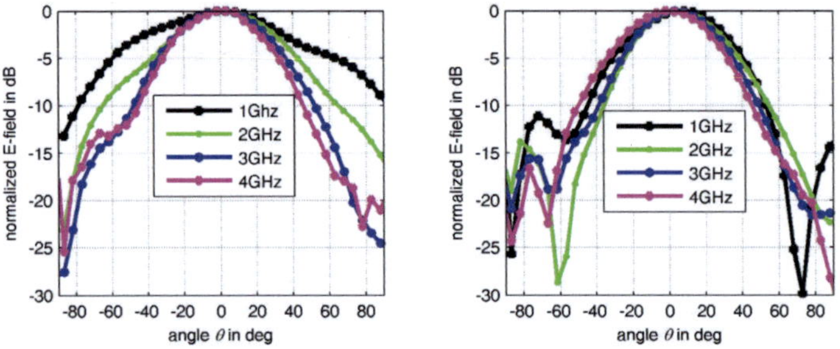

(a) H-Plane (b) E-Plane

Fig. 6.5: Measured radiation pattern of the Bowtie antenna in PEG solution.

6.3 UWB imaging system for breast cancer detection

In this section, the performance of the broadband Bowtie antenna is experimentally evaluated. The antenna is used inside a hemispherical array for the detection of tumor in a synthesized breast-mimicking phantom. In the following the near-field imaging system including the measurement setup for collecting the scattered signals and the breast phantoms are presented.

6.3.1 Measurement setup for breast phantom imaging

To realize a realistic setup having the potential of being later employed in clinical trials, a 16 element hemispherical array was implemented (see Fig. 6.6). The hemispherical arrangement is known to outperform the cylindrical array regarding the imaging performance ([9]). As explained in the previous section, the Bowtie antennas were designed to work between two media; i.e. the radiating Bowtie was in contact to a breast-mimicking phantom whereas the feeding network was kept inside a low-permittivity medium (preferably air). With that in mind, for the laboratory setup, a polystyrene hemisphere was chosen as the base of the array. The dielectric properties of polystyrene were very close to those of air, making it a good medium for the background in the initial laboratory implementation. The hemisphere had an inner radius of 5.45 cm.

To arrange 16 antennas on a hemispherical surface, two important criteria were considered: the antenna elements were positioned so that the adjacent elements were as equi-distant as possible. Moreover, as it was discussed in [33], to have a good cross range resolution, it was preferred to arrange the antenna elements in a rectangular form. Having considered these two criteria, the final arrangement of the array displayed in Fig. 6.6 was chosen.

The E8363B vector network analyzer (VNA) from Agilent Technologies was used as the RF transmitter and reciever. The output power of VNA was 5 dBm, the IF-Bandwidth was set to 300 Hz and 1601 points were considered in the bandwidth from 1 to 7.5 GHz. Furthermore, a power amplifier of approximately 11 dB gain was connected to the VNA output leading to a final output power of around 16 dBm. For the collection of signals, a multistatic scenario was adopted and the antenna elements of the array acted sequentially as transmitter while all the other antennas acted as receiver (Rx). A programmable RF mechanical switch matrix was used to automatically connect each Tx-Rx antenna-pair to the VNA, resulting in 240 different measurements, half of which were considered for the imaging due to the reciprocity. A sketch of the near-field imaging system together with a picture of the implemented imaging system are shown in Fig. 6.7.

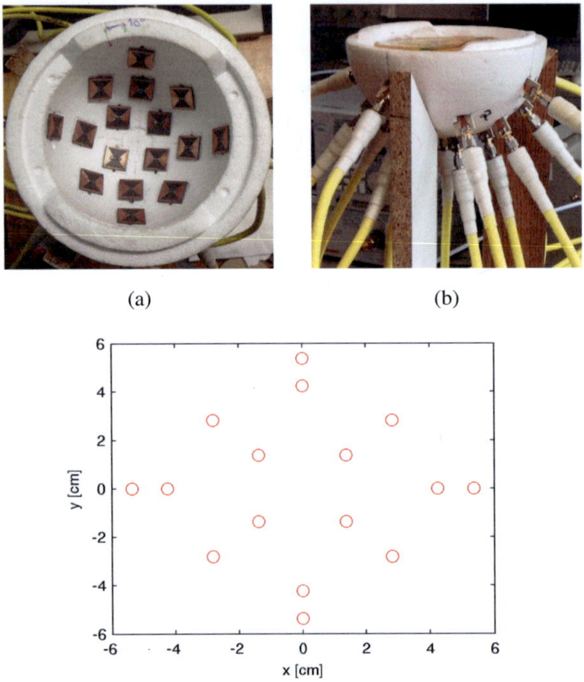

(a) (b)

(c)

Fig. 6.6: (a) and (b) Array configuration on a styropor base; (c) the 2D mapped positions of the antenna elements.

6.3.2 Synthesized breast phantoms

For the evaluation of the proposed near-field imaging system, a hemispherical breast phantom of radius 5.45 cm was built. The breast phantom was a mixture of water (47%), sugar (47%) and gelatin (6%). The tumor phantom was approximately 10 mm in diameter and was made up of the same ingredients, however with the following proportions: water (71%), sugar (14.5%) and gelatin (14.5%) (Fig. 6.8).

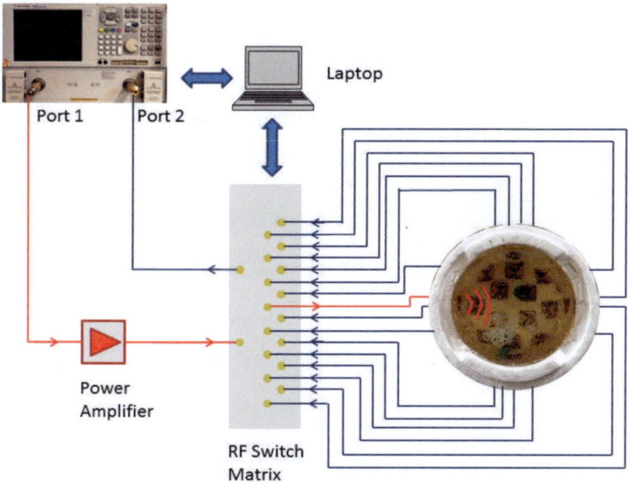

(a)

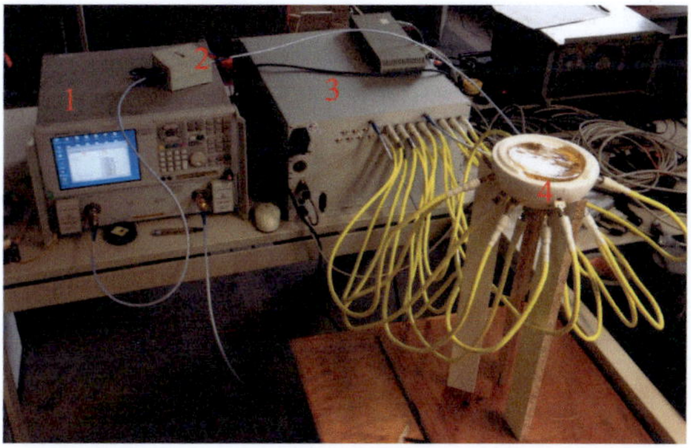

(b)

Fig. 6.7: (a) Schematic of the imaging system; (b) the actual implemented near-field imaging system: 1: VNA, 2: power amplifier, 3: mechanical swich matrix, 4: antenna array with breast phantom inside.

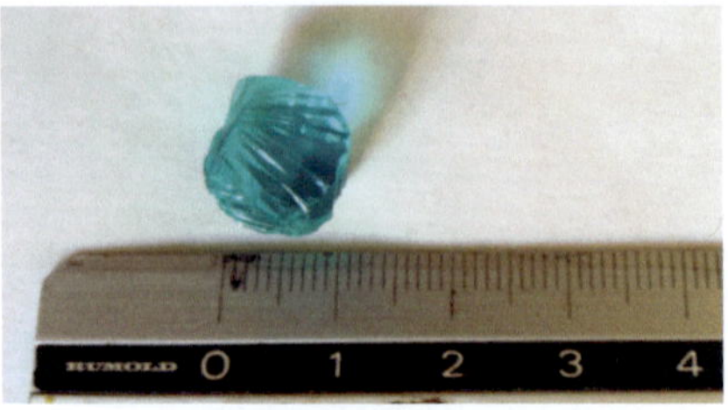

Fig. 6.8: Tumor phantom approximately 10 mm in diameter

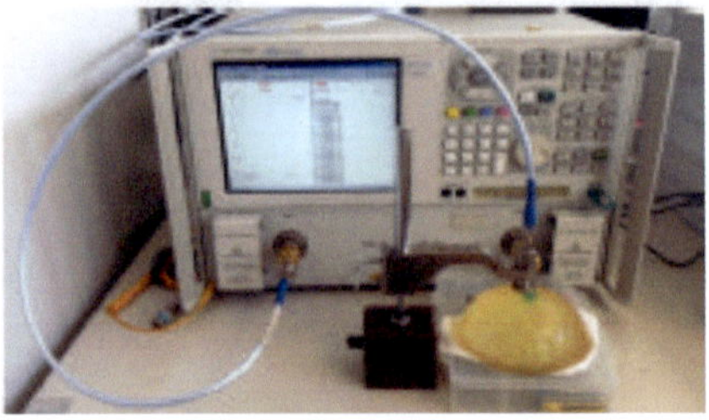

Fig. 6.9: Measurement setup for the characterization of the dielectric properties of the breast phantom.

The permittivity and conductivity of the breast phantom and tumor were measured using the Agilent Dielectric Probe Kit (85070E)(Fig. 6.9) and were compared to the corresponding values predicted by the Cole - Cole formula [30] in Fig. 6.10. As shown in the figure, the measured values for the breast phantom were between the high and average adipose categories of normal breast. The synthesized phantoms with one and two tumors are displayed in Fig. 6.11.

6.3.3 Radar beamforming algorithm

For the image reconstruction, a beamforming Radar approach has been used. The signals are measured in the frequency domain following a multistatic scenario. The recorded signals are afterwards filtered (Tuckey window) and converted

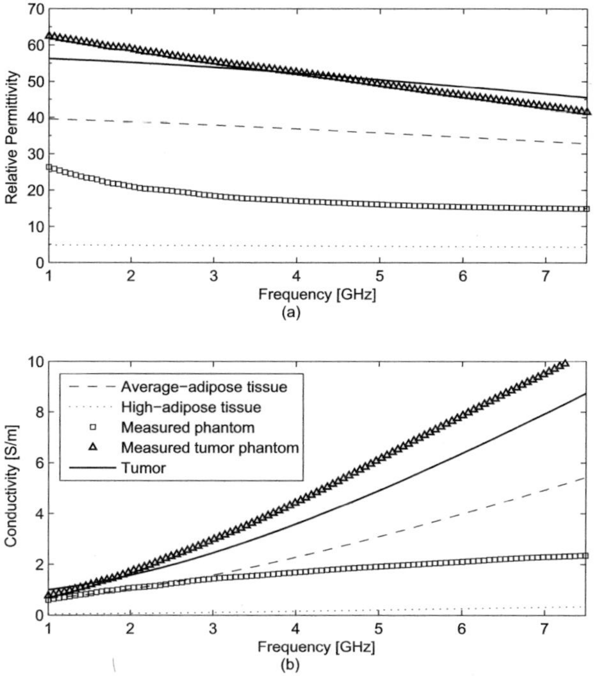

Fig. 6.10: Relative permittivity and conductivity of normal breast tissue and tumor as obtained from the Cole-Cole equation [16] compared to the measured dielectric properties of the synthesized breast phantom; (a) relative permittivity, (b) conductivity.

into time domain using IFFT. In the following, the imaging algorithms will be reviewed.

Conventional Delay and Sum

The Delay and Sum (DAS) beamformer is a passive process doing exactly what its name implies; that is, the recorded scattered signals are first assigned appropriate time delays so that the beamformer will focus on a specific point inside the target. Afterwards the time-aligned signals are added and the energy of the resulting signal is estimated which corresponds to the intensity level of a single focal point within the target (see Fig. 6.12). The output of a DAS beamformer can be explicitly represented as follows:

$$Z[n, r_0] = \sum_{i=1}^{M} X_i[n - \tau_{id}(r_0)] \tag{6.1}$$

where $\tau_{id}(r_0) = \tau_{max} - round[\tau_i(r_0).f_s]$.
M is the total number of the received signals ($X_i[n]$'s). $\tau_i(r_0)$ is the round-trip distance from the corresponding transmit and receive antennas to the focus point r_0, fs is the sampling frequency and τ_{max} is the maximum delay.

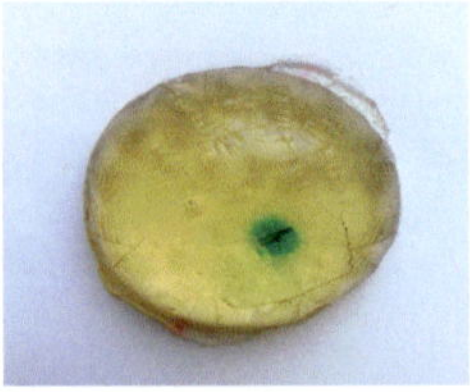

(a) 1 tumor: view from the top

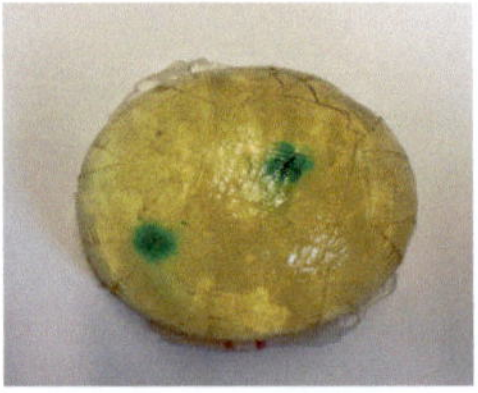

(b) 2 tumors: view from the top

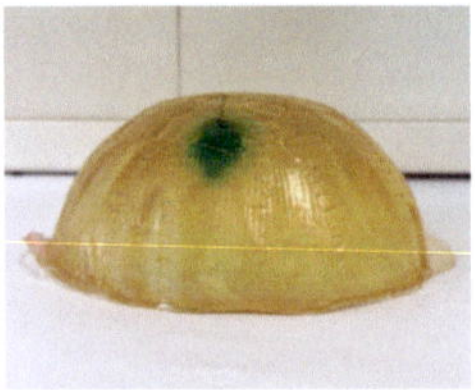

(c) 1 tumor: side view

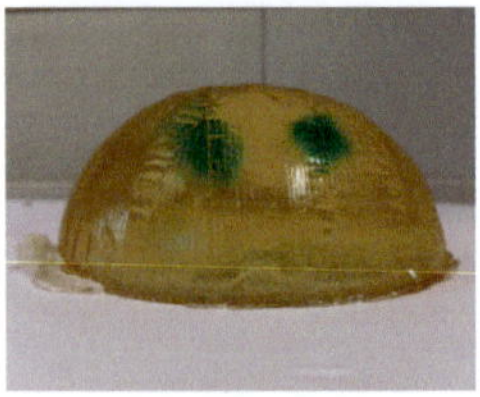

(d) 2 tumors: side view

Fig. 6.11: The synthesized breast phantoms of (a) and (c) one tumor and (b) and (d) two tumors (left and right columns, respectively).

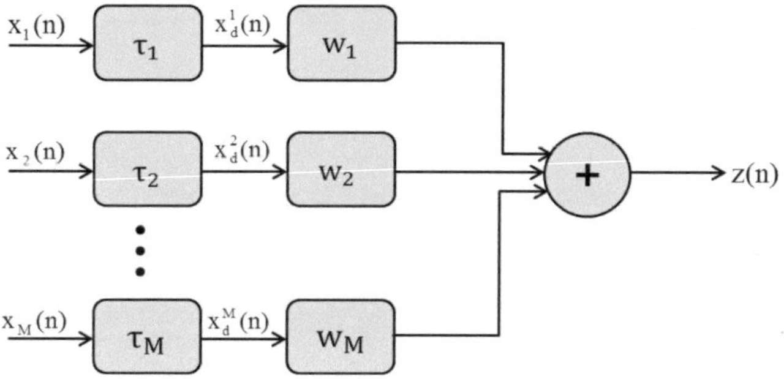

Fig. 6.12: The block diagram of a conventional delay-and-sum beamformer.

The final step would be to estimate the energy level of the beamformer output for each focal point; this is done as follows:

$$I[r_0] = \sum_{i=1}^{N} |Z[i, r_0]|^2 \tag{6.2}$$

N is the total number of samples.

By adjusting appropriate time delays, all the points within the target volume will be scanned and as a result an image will be reconstructed. Although in principal no windowing is necessarily performed in the conventional DAS, here in this research the delayed signals ($X_d^i(n)$ in Fig. 6.12) are first windowed using Hamming window coefficients and the resulting signals are afterwards added together.

Considering the fact that the delays can be implemented either in time or frequency domain, the technique proves to be efficient for both narrowband and broadband applications. However, although the beamformer has several advantages the most important of which are simplicity and robustness, its performance is limited in terms of artifact removal and resolution.

To tackle the problems of the conventional DAS and enhance the performance of the beamformer, the output of the beamformer ($z(n)$ in Fig. 6.12) is once again windowed using coherence factor windowing coefficients.

Enhanced DAS using Coherence Factor Coefficients

Coherence factor (CF) coefficients are defined as the ratio of the coherent sum of the delayed signals to the ratio of the non-coherent sum of the delayed signals [55]; (unitless quantity varying from zero to one); it means:

$$CF(n) = \frac{\left|\sum_{m=1}^{M} X_d^m(n)\right|^2}{M \sum_{m=1}^{M} \left|X_d^m(n)\right|^2} \tag{6.3}$$

$X_d[n]$ refers to the delayed signal. These coefficients can be interpreted as a measure of the coherency of the recorded signals coming from a given point inside the imaging area. By taking these coefficients into account, the directivity of the beamformer will be considerably increased and the effect can be directly observed in the increased dynamic range of the system, signal to clutter ratio as well as the significant improvement in the resolution of the detection. This is mainly due to the fact that the clutter signal is of low coherency whereas at the points where a strong scatterer exists, a high coherency will be measured.
To apply the CF coefficients no pre-knowledge of the scene (e.g. number of scatteres) is required. The coefficients are estimated from the delayed signals and they are applied to the output of the beamformer (to the final windowed signals). The estimation of the coefficients and applying them to the signal adds no extra computational cost to the system.
The output of the beamformer after applying the CF coefficients will be:

$$Z_{out}[n, r_0] = CF(n).Z[n, r_0] \tag{6.4}$$

The energy of this signal will be then estimated which would correspond to the intensity value of the image regarding the focus point r_0.

In the following, the imaging results obtained using the UWB imaging system will be presented and discussed.

6.4 Measured imaging results and discussion

As explained previously, using a UWB antenna array consisting of 16 elements (Fig. 6.3 and Fig. 6.6) and the breast phantoms shown in Fig. 6.11, 120 signals in frequency range of 1.2 - 7 GHz were recorded. For data calibration, since we were only interested in the response of the tumor, a second measurement was performed with the array being 15 degree rotated and the resultant signals were subtracted correspondingly [27]. This allows for removal of unwanted signals such as those due to antenna coupling and skin reflection. The tumor response will appear at different times in each of the two measurements, further enabling tumor localization. The calibrated signals were afterwards transformed into time domain and fed into the UWB image reconstruction unit based on the enhanced Delay-and-Sum algorithm.

6.4.1 Breast phantom with one-tumor

In the first measurement, the breast phantom with one tumor of 1.3 cm diameter and at a depth of approximately 2 cm (off-center) was placed inside the measurement system of Fig. 6.7. The calibrated signals were processed in the reconstruction unit and in Fig. 6.13 the corresponding imaging results are displayed (all the imaging results present the 2D slices of the relative energy map of the output of the beamformer). Compared to the pictures of the phantom in Fig. 6.11 (a) and (c), it was observed that the tumor was successfully detected in the 3D space at the correct position in both x-y and x-z planes however with a different resolution. This was already expected, since the effective size of the array in the two views was different, thus leading to a different resolution. For a more quantitative look at the tumor response, in Fig. 6.14 and 6.15 image cuts at the position of tumor are presented.

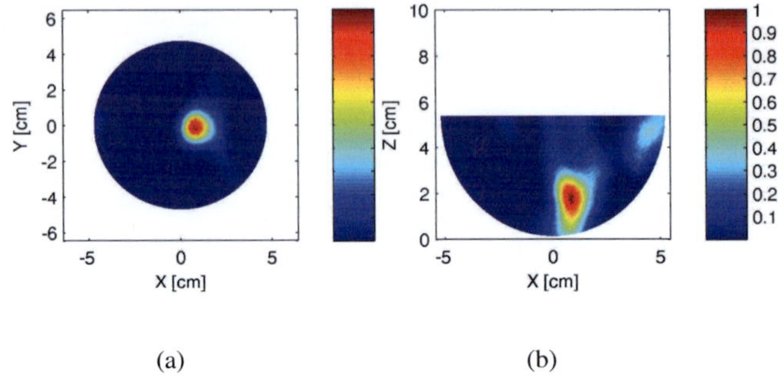

Fig. 6.13: The imaging results of the one-tumor breast phantom in (a) horizontal (x-y) and (b) vertical (x-z) planes (linear scale).

6.4.2 Breast phantom with two-tumors

For the second evaluation of the proposed measurement system, the phantom of Fig. 6.11 (b) and (d) with two embedded tumors of different size and at different depths was used. One of the tumors had a diameter of approximately 1 cm and was located at a depth of 1.8 cm. The second tumor was 1.5 cm in diameter and 3 cm deep inside the breast phantom.

The image in Fig. 6.16 corresponds to the stacked x-y plane image when looking at the phantom from above (i.e. all the images in the z-direction are added together). In this image, it is possible to recognize the two tumors: one approximately in the center and the other nearly 4.5 cm above it. The reconstructed positions agree quite well to the real positions of the tumors.

To detect the depth of each tumor, we looked at the reconstructed images at different z (horizontal) layers. In Fig. 6.17 and 6.18, the images of 6 vertical planes are shown. The first three sub-figures corresponding to z= 0.1 cm to z= 2 cm, show the first tumor near the center (z= 0 points to the base of the phantom). The other three sub-figures, z= 3 cm to z= 5 cm, mainly include the second tumor that was located near the surface of the phantom. In Fig. 6.18(c) refering

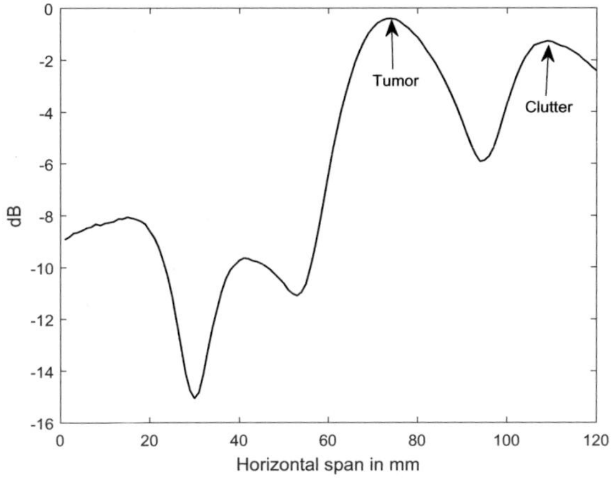

(a)

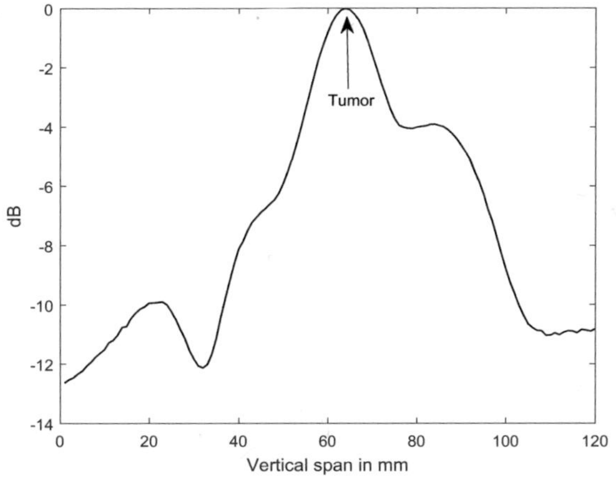

(b)

Fig. 6.14: Image-cuts at the position of tumor in the measurement result of Fig. 6.13 (a); (a) horizontal cut, (b) vertical cut.

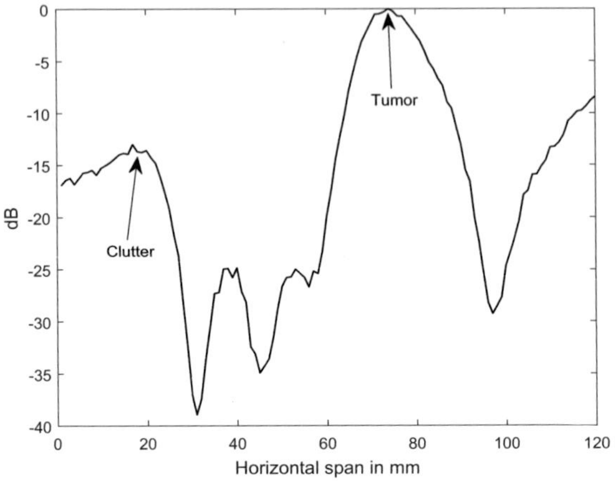

(a)

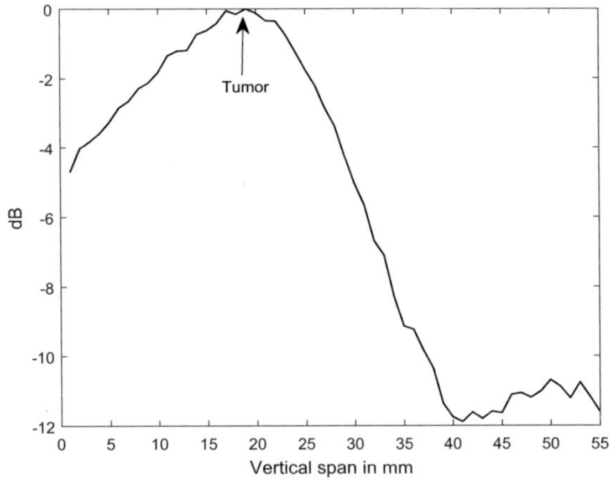

(b)

Fig. 6.15: Image-cuts at the position of tumor in the measurement result of Fig. 6.13 (b); (a) horizontal cut, (b) vertical cut.

Tabelle 6.1: signal to clutter ratio (SCR) and position of tumors (x y z) in cm

Breast Phantom	SCR	Actual tumor position	Detected tumor position
with one tumor	4 dB	(1.2, -1, 2)	(1, -0.1, 1.8)
with two tumors-tumor no.I	4.7 dB	(0.6, 3.4, 1.8)	(-0.2, 4, 2)
with two tumors-tumor no.II	3.5 dB	(0.8, -1, 3)	(0, -0.2, 3)

to the image of the phantom near the breast-air interface in the uppermost layer, a relative large artifact is present that was due to the large reflections at the interface. Some quantitative results regarding the performance of the system are reported in Table 6.1. By comparing the actual position and depth of the tumors to the detected ones, it can be concluded that all the tumors were successfully detected in 3D space.

Therefore, the proposed miniaturized Bowtie was successfully evaluated for detecting tumor phantoms in a breast mimicking phantom having dielectric properties similar to average adipose breast tissues. The antenna is a very efficient radiating element covering a broad range of low and high operational frequencies compared to the other structures so far proposed for breast cancer detection.

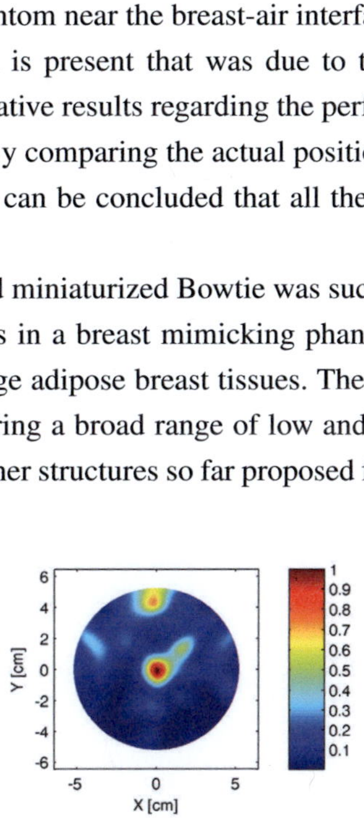

Fig. 6.16: The stacked image of the breast phantom with two tumors in horizontal plane (x-y).

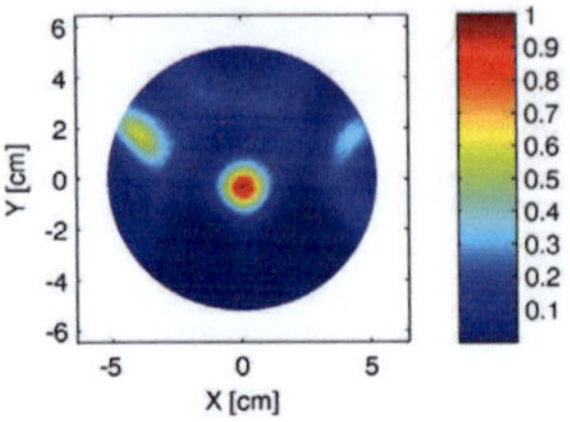

(a)

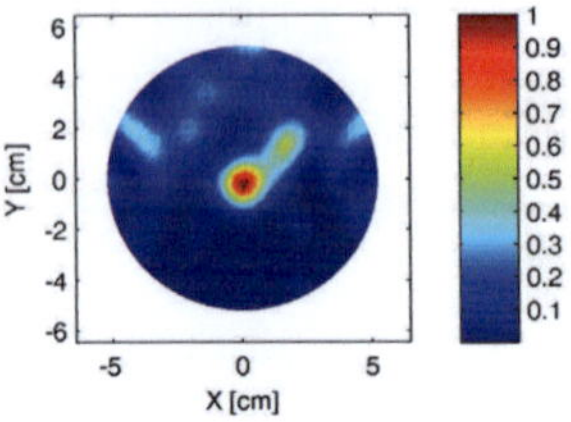

(b)

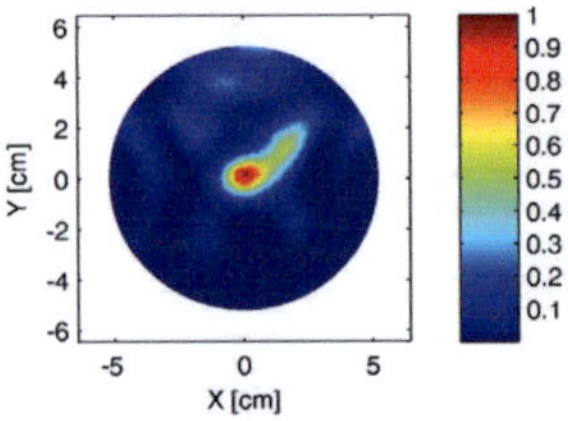

(c)

Fig. 6.17: The imaging results corresponding to the two-tumor breast phantom at different horizontal layers (z-axis); (a) z= 0.1 cm, (b) z= 1 cm and (c) z= 2 cm.

6.5 Planar Bowtie antenna for head imaging

As for the head imaging application, in the previous chapters the microwave tomography approach was introduced as one efficient alternative approach to conventional techniques. The Radar approach applied to breast imaging in this chapter can in principle be applied to head imaging as well. Although in this case more challenge is expected due to the high contrast of the dielectric properties of head tissues and as a result the applicability of the technique to this target application has to be carefully examined. Specially in case of hemorrhagic stroke, due to the higher dielectric properties of the affected regions compared to the

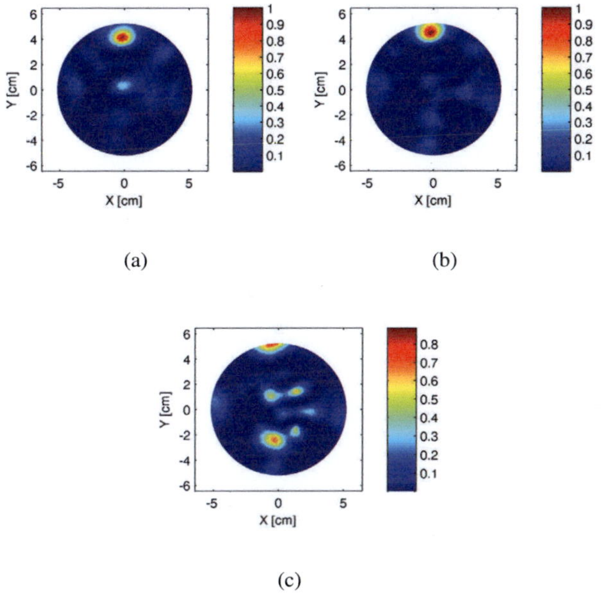

Fig. 6.18: The imaging results corresponding to the two-tumor breast phantom at different horizontal layers (z-axis); (a) z= 3 cm, (b) z= 4 cm and (c) z= 5 cm.

surrounding tissues, the Radar technique is expected to be efficient in detecting the damaged area due to the stroke.

In [48] a rather similar technique is used for stroke detection however with a 2D antenna array. In that research, the antennas are not optimized for biomedical applications ([43], [42] and [59]) and specially for head imaging and they are simply placed in some distance to the head phantom in air. Regarding the high contrast of the air and the head tissues as discussed in Chapter 3 this leads to a considerable loss of energy at the interface between air to skin and as a result the overall imaging performance is degraded.

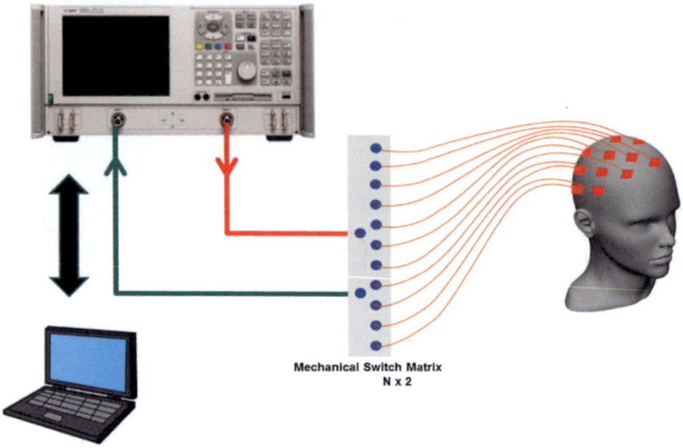

Fig. 6.19: The imaging setup for head imaging via Radar beamforming approach.

In this section some preliminary results are presented in order to introduce the idea behind using the modified Bowtie antenna in a Radar-based imaging system for head imaging. It must be emphasized that some more in deep investigation regarding the applicability and efficiency of this approach for head imaging is required.

6.5.1 Imaging setup for the detection of stroke

A sketch of the imaging system is shown in Fig. 6.19. With the help of a mechanical switch matrix, it is possible to switch between the antenna elements of the conformal array in a multistatic scenario to obtain scattering signals from all over the head phantom (the same imaging procedure as in the previous section for the detection of tumor in breast-mimicking phantoms).
The Bowtie antenna was introduced in Chapter 4 for application in 3D microwave tomography. The same Bowtie antenna with the bandwidth of 0.8-3 GHz and its planar structure can be also considered as an efficient structure for head imaging via microwave Radar beamforming. The conformal structure of the antenna

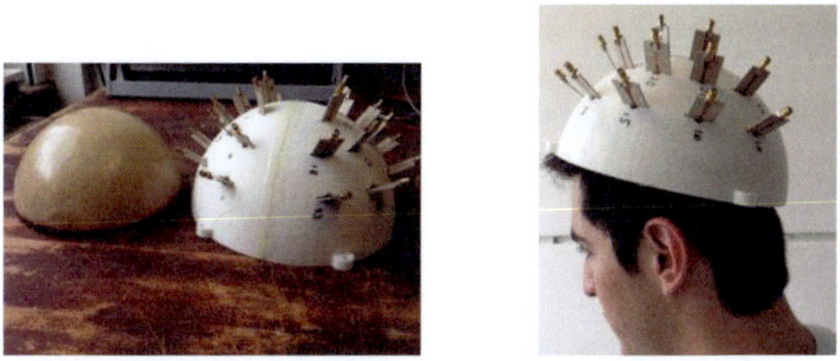

(a) (b)

Fig. 6.20: The planar Bowtie antennas arranged inside a hemispherical array-base for head imaging.

with its directional radiation assist in efficient coupling of microwave signals into the head.

In the following, the Bowtie antenna is used inside a helmet-shaped array base (Styrofoam) to be worn by the patient (Fig. 6.20). In an initial investigation, the antenna elements were divided into two groups of each 12 elements (all together 24 elements) and each group was positioned in one half of the hemisphere-shaped array base to cover one half of the brain (phantom).

A multilayer head phantom composing of four layers representing similar dielectric properties to skin, skull, gray matter and white matter developed in the Institute of Biomedical Engineering (IBT) at KIT was used during the imaging as the target (Fig. 6.21). A stroke phantom with approximate blood properties (sphere of 2 cm diameter) was inside the gray matter region. The phantom was placed inside the hemispherical array and as a very initial investigation, a monostatic approach was used to collect 24 broadband signals in the frequency range of 0.8-3 GHz.

6.5.2 Monostatic Radar approach for focusing the stroke response

The image reconstruction algorithm was the modified delay and sum algorithm applied in the previous section for breast phantom imaging. However, the pre-processing of the recorded signal in order to focus the response of the stroke region and to get rid of the other unwanted contributions from all the other layers other than stroke was different (the so called data calibration technique).

Data calibration for extracting the stroke response

As for data calibration in order to extract the sole response of the stroke region, considering that a stroke existed only in one half of the hemisphere and regarding the mostly symmetrical shape of the left-side and right-side parts of the head phantom (in fact actual human head) the signals recorded by 12 antennas on one side were used as the reference signals and were subtracted from the other 12 recorded signals on the other side. Considering the symmetry of the two parts of the brain the main difference in the recorded signals will come from the stroke region [48].

Measured imaging results with head-mimicking phantom

The measured monostatic results are presented in Fig. 6.22. The stroke region has been detected in both horizontal and vertical planes at the correct position. The relatively high clutter and noise present in the figures can be reduced by applying a multistatic approach and an enhanced array design with more antenna elements with more efficient distribution of the elements.
Therefore, considering the example applications of breast imaging and head imaging in this chapter, the modified Bowtie antenna can be regarded as an efficient broadband planar structure to be used in conformal arrays for 3D biomedical applications.

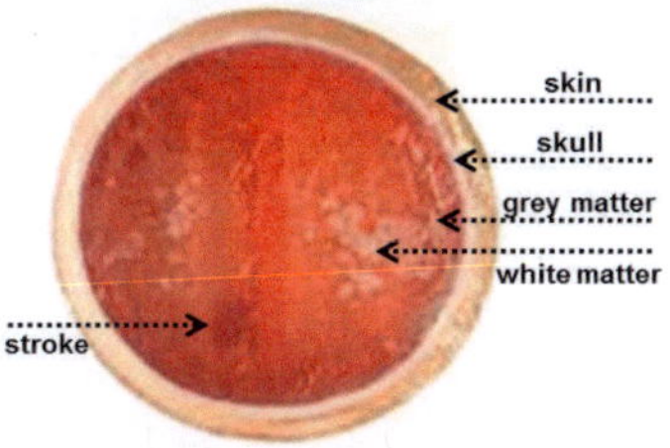

(a)

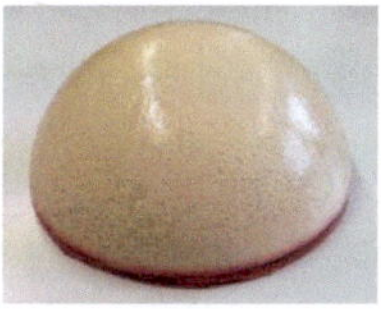

(b)

Fig. 6.21: The multilayer head-mimicking phantom (developed in the Institute of Biomedical Engineering (IBT) - KIT).

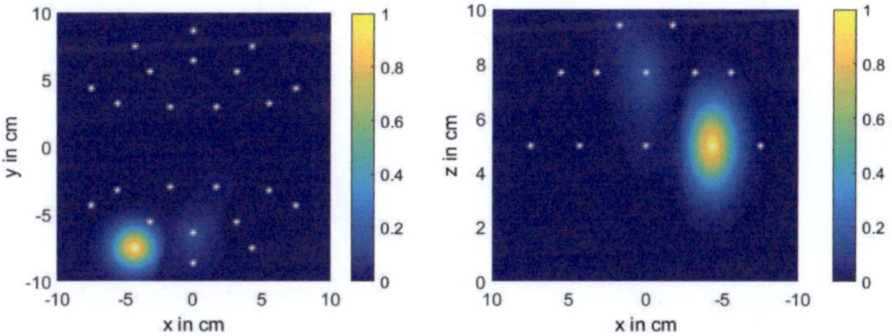

(a) (b)

Fig. 6.22: The measured monostatic imaging results; (a) stacked vertical layers x-y, (b) stacked horizontal layers x-z.

7 Conclusion and future work

This work dealt with some concerns regarding antenna design for microwave medical imaging applications. It was discussed that the design of an antenna structure for microwave medical imaging is very much dependent on the target application as well as the exploited imaging technique.
Broadband antennas were proposed for microwave medical imaging and several criteria were introduced for the evaluation of the performance of antenna structures for different imaging methods. It was discussed that depending on the exploited imaging technique, different specification of the antennas are required. Therefore, before proposing an antenna structure for application in microwave medical imaging, it is necessary to discuss the required antenna characteristic and accordingly to proceed with antenna design. Three microwave imaging techniques were considered and after discussing the antenna requirement of each technique, efficient structures were proposed for each imaging method. The performance of the antennas were evaluated inside imaging systems for stroke detection and breast cancer detection as example applications.
The following sections include a summary of the achievements of this work and some suggestions for the future extension of the current research.

7.1 Conclusion

The required specification of an antenna for microwave medical imaging is dependent on the target application. After studying the interaction of microwave signals to a multilayer head model as an example application, a proper frequency range was proposed for human head imaging in chapter 3. An anatomically realistic MRI-derived 2D head model with an embedded stroke region was successfully reconstructed using microwave tomography at a single frequency within the proposed optimum range. The nonlinear iterative Gauss-Newton algorithm was applied to the scattered electric fields recorded at 24 points around the model and in a blind reconstruction the dielectric map of the numerical model and the stroke region were successfully reconstructed. The results motivate the application of microwave imaging (tomographic approach) for the detection of stroke in human head.

After demonstrating the potential of microwave imaging for the detection of stroke as a relatively new emerging application, the rest of the work focused on designing high-performance antennas for practical imaging systems and proposing efficient criteria for the evaluation of the performance of the antennas prior to performing imaging.

The antenna requirements for 3D microwave tomography were discussed in chapter 4 and a modified Bowtie antenna featuring a broad bandwidth and compact dimension was proposed for this imaging method. The broadband response was obtained by connecting the two arms of the Bowtie thereby enabling the antenna operation from 0.8 GHz to 3 GHz. The short-connected arms further resulted in miniaturization of the antenna and decrease of the lower frequency of operation. The antenna characteristic when fed by a balun structure was shown to be reasonably similar to an ideal discrete port feeding. Therefore, for the modeling of the antenna in a 3D numerical forward solver, the antenna can be efficiently represented only by the radiating element. This would significantly reduce the complexity of the forward solver model without sacrificing the accuracy. The antenna was compared to the relatively simple monopole antenna so far widely used in microwave tomography imaging systems.

An alternative procedure to the computationally extensive full-wave 3D microwave tomography is the synthetic 3D microwave tomography approach. Criteria were proposed for the evaluation of the optimum antenna structure for synthetic 3D microwave tomography in chapter 5. The performances of two antennas were examined and compared for application in this imaging technique. The previously designed Bowtie antenna was compared to a Vivaldi structure regarding the operational bandwidth, efficiency of the antenna when modeled as a point source in a 2D numerical solver and finally the coupled power into a phantom. It turned out that despite of the better matching of the Bowtie antenna in the whole frequency range, the Vivaldi antenna outperformed the Bowtie antenna regarding the modeling error when the antenna was modeled as a point-source in the 2D forward solver of MEEP.

To validate the proposed criteria, two imaging scenarios were simulated in the commercial software CST. Two antenna arrays (Bowtie array and Vivaldi array) surrounded a multilayer head model and following a multistatic scenario scattering signals were recorded in each imaging setup. Using the nonlinear iterative Gauss-Newton algorithm, the dielectric map of the head model was successfully reconstructed at 1 GHz using the Vivaldi array. A stroke area deep inside the white matter was detected in both permittivity and conductivity profiles. As for the Bowtie array, the high modeling error predicted by the proposed criteria led to poor reconstructed imaging results. It was mentioned that the synthetic approach can alternatively be used to accelerate full-wave 3D microwave tomography by providing an initial approximation of the dielectric properties of the IO.

Another widely exploited imaging technique is the qualitative Radar approach that works well for detecting targets with high dielectric contrast relative to the surrounding tissues (e.g. tumor detection in breast). This imaging technique was discussed in chapter 6. For the application of breast cancer detection using the microwave Radar approach, the design of a compact antenna element with large fractional bandwidth covering both low and high frequencies to ensure good penetration as well as high resolution is a big challenge. In this research, an efficient compact Bowtie antenna with the largest dimension of 15 mm and a bandwidth of 1.2-7 GHz was proposed for UWB near-field breast imaging and it was characterized via simulations and measurements.

The antenna was used inside a hemispherical array of 16 elements for the detection of tumors in synthesized breast mimicking phantoms. The implemented near-field imaging system was evaluated using two average-adipose breast phantoms with one and two embedded tumors respectively. The successful detection of the tumors in the 3D space proved the efficiency and potential of the proposed UWB imaging system for breast cancer detection.

The Radar approach was further used for head imaging as well. Although this application is more complicated compared to breast imaging, the initial measurement results using an array of Bowtie antennas surrounding a multilayer head phantom showed the potential of the technique for head imaging. In the reconstructed images, the stroke region modeled as blood seemed to be detectable as a dominant scattering region inside the phantom.

All in all, as discussed in this dissertation, microwaves are sensitive to the difference of the dielectric properties of the tissues. In competition to the available imaging techniques, microwave's only chance is to provide significant advantages regarding cost, portability, simple installation and performance. It was discussed that the antenna array design has a direct impact on the final image quality. Some challenges regarding the optimum antenna structure for different microwave medical imaging techniques were addressed in this research.

7.2 Future extension of the current research

The research performed in this work can be extended in several directions:

The Bowtie antenna proposed for application in full-wave 3D microwave tomography in chapter 4 can be utilized in a 3D imaging scenario (simulation and/or measurement) with and without modeling the feeding taper in the numerical simulation. The imaging results will be then compared to those obtained by an array of monopole antennas. The comparison will be regarding the computational time and the imaging efficiency.

Another complementary research would be the implementation of the proposed Vivaldi antenna in an experimental imaging system for synthetic 3D or full-wave

3D microwave tomography. An initial step in synthetic 3D microwave tomography would be the optimization of the antenna array and the imaging tank (dimension of the tank and the position of the antennas on the walls of the tank) using the criteria proposed for the minimization of the modeling error. The proposed criteria also help choosing the best frequencies with minimum modeling error. As mentioned before, the optimization of the imaging system prior to performing actual imaging would save a lot of computational time and assist in further improving the efficiency of the imaging system.

Further extension of the current research can be improving the imaging results quantitatively. For instance, in this work it was shown that microwave tomography has a good potential for stroke detection (imaging results of a 2D MRI-derived head mode). In the imaging scenario, although the stroke was clearly detected in both permittivity and conductivity profiles at 1 GHz, the quantitative dielectric properties of the reconstructed tissues need to be improved. This issue is especially of great importance in practical applications in order to distinguish between ischemic and hemorrhagic stroke. The quantitative results can be improved in several ways. One way would be to use a frequency hopping technique to take advantage of both the low and high frequency spectrum. This way the imaging results at lower frequencies serve as the starting guess at higher frequencies and step by step the resolution and quantitative results will improve. In a similar way, the reconstructed imaging results obtained using the Vivaldi array in Chapter 5 can be improved using the frequency hopping technique. The large bandwidth of the proposed Vivaldi antenna would allow the incremental change in the frequency in this case to improve the results quantitatively.

The applicability of the Radar beamforming technique to head imaging needs to be further investigated. For this purpose an enhanced antenna array design and applying a multistatic scenario for a more efficient focusing of the stroke area is recommended. The applicability of the technique needs to be examined by attempting to localize stroke phantoms in different locations inside white matter and grey matter tissue-mimicking phantoms.

Bibliography

[1] AL-JOUMAYLY, M. A. ; AGUILAR, S. M. ; BEHDAD, N. ; HAGNESS, S. C.: Dual-band miniaturized patch antennas for microwave breast imaging. In: *IEEE Anten. and Wireless Propag. lett.* 9 (2010), S. 268–271

[2] BALANIS, C. A.: Antenna Theory: Analysis and Design. In: *Wiley* (2005)

[3] BOLOMEY, J. ; JOFRE, L.: Three decades of active microwave imaging achievements, difficulties and future challenges. In: *Proc. ICWITS* (2010)

[4] BOND, E. J. ; LI, X. ; HAGNESS, S. C. ; VEEN, B. D. V.: Microwave imaging via space-time beamforming for early detection of breast cancer. In: *IEEE Trans. Antennas Propag.* 51 (2003), Nr. 8, S. 1690 –1705

[5] BRANDSTATTER, B. ; HOLLAUS, K. ; HUTTEN, H. ; MAYER, M. ; MERWA, R. ; ; SCHARFETTER, H.: Direct estimation of Cole parameters in multifrequency EIT using a regularized Gauss-Newton method. In: *Physiol. Meas.* 24 (2003), Nr. 2, S. 437–448

[6] BULYSHEV, A. E. ; SEMENOV, S. Y. ; SOUVOROV, A. E. ; SVENSON, R. H. ; NAZAROV, A. G. ; SIZOV, Y. E. ; TATSIS, G. P.: Computational modeling of three-dimensional microwave tomography of breast cancer. In: *Physiol. Meas.* 48 (2001), Nr. 9, S. 1053–1056

[7] BURFEINDT, M. J. ; BEHDAD, N. ; VEEN, B. D. V. ; HAGNESS, S. C.: Quantitative microwave imaging of realistic numerical breast phantoms using an enclosed array of multiband, miniaturized patch antennas. In: *IEEE Antennas Wireless Propag. Lett.* 11 (2012), S. 1626–1629

[8] CHANDRA, R. ; ZHOU, H. ; BALASINGHAM, I. ; NARAYANAN, R. M.: On the Opportunities and Challenges in Microwave Medical Sensing and Imaging. In: *IEEE Trans. Biomedical Eng.* 62 (2015), S. 1667–1682

[9] D. KURRANT, C. Curtis E. F. J. Bourqui B. J. Bourqui: Evaluation of 3-D Acquisition Surfaces for Radar-Based Microwave Breast Imaging. In: *IEEE Trans. on Antennas Propag.* 63 (2015), S. 4910–4920

[10] DAVIS, S. K. ; TANDRADINATA, H. ; HAGNESS, S. C. ; VEEN, B. D. V.: Ultrawideband microwave breast cancer detection: A detection-theoretic approach using the generalized likelihood ratio test. In: *IEEE Trans. Biomed. Eng.* 52 (2005), Nr. 7, S. 1237–1250

[11] ELAHI, M. A. ; SHAHZAD, A. ; GLAVIN, M. ; JONES, E. ; O'HALLORAN, M.: Hybrid Artifact Removal for Confocal Microwave Breast Imaging. In: *IEEE Anten. and Wireless Propag. lett.* 13 (2014), S. 149–152

[12] FANG, Q. ; MEANEY, P. M. ; PAULSEN, K. D.: Singular value analysis of the Jacobian matrix in microwave image reconstruction. In: *IEEE Trans. on Antennas Propag.* 54 (2006), Nr. 8, S. 2371–2380

[13] FEAR, E. C. ; HAGNESS, S. C. ; MEANEY, P. M. ; OKONIEWSKI, M. ; STUCHLY, M. A.: Enhancing breast tumor detection with nearfield imaging. In: *IEEE Microw. Mag.* 3 (2002), S. 48–56

[14] FEAR, E. C. ; LI, X. ; HAGNESS, S. C. ; STUCHLY, M. A.: Confocal microwave imaging for breast cancer detection: Localization of tumors in three dimensions. In: *IEEE Trans. Biomed. Eng.* 49 (2002), Nr. 8, S. 812–822

[15] FEAR, E. C. ; MEANEY, P. M. ; STUCHLY, M. A.: Microwave for breast cancer detection? In: *IEEE Potentials* 22 (2003), S. 12–18

[16] GABRIEL, S. ; LAU, R. W. ; GABRIEL, C.: The dielectric properties of biological tissues: III. parametric models for the dielectric spectrum of tissues. In: *Phys. Med. Biol.* 41 (1996), S. 2271–2293

[17] GILMORE, C. ; ZAKARIA, A. ; MOJABI, P. ; OSTADRAHIMI, M. ; PISTORIUS, S. ; VETRI, J. L.: The University of Manitoba Microwave Imaging Repository: A Two-Dimensional Microwave Scattering Database for Testing Inversion and Calibration Algorithms [Measurements Corner]. In: *IEEE Antennas and Propag. Magazine* 53 (2011), S. 126 – 133

[18] GOLNABI, A. H. ; MEANEY, P. M. ; PAULSEN, K. D.: Tomographic microwave imaging with incorporated prior spatial information. In: *IEEE Trans. Microw. Tech.* 39 (2013), S. 2129–2136

[19] GRZEGORCZYK, T. ; MEANEY, P. ; KAUFMAN, P. ; ALEXANDER, R. di-Florio ; PAULSEN, K.: Fast 3-D tomographic microwave imaging for breast cancer detection. In: *IEEE Transaction on medical imaging* 31 (2012), Nr. 8, S. 1584 –1592

[20] GUARDIOLA, M. ; JOFRE, L. ; CAPDEVILA, S. ; ROMEU, J.: UWB brain differential imaging capabilities. In: *Proc. Eucap* (2012)

[21] GUO, L. ; ABBOSH, A. M.: Optimization-Based Confocal Microwave Imaging in Medical Applications. In: *IEEE Trans. on Antennas and Propag.* 63 (2015), S. 3531–3539

[22] JOACHIMOWICZ, N. ; PICHOT, C. ; HUGONIN, J. P.: Inverse scattering: an iterative numerical method for electromagnetic imaging. In: *IEEE Trans. Antennas Propagat.* 39 (1991), S. 1742–1753

[23] JR., H. P. A. ; ZOPPO, G. del ; ALBERTS, M. J.: Guidelines for the early management of adults with ischemic stroke. In: *Stroke* 38 (2007), S. 1655–1711

[24] KELLNBERGER, S. ; HAJIABOLI, A. ; RAZANSKY, D. ; NTZIACHRISTOS, V.: Near-field thermoacoustic tomography of small animals. In: *Phys. Med. Biol.* 56 (2011), S. 3433–3444

[25] KLEMM, M. ; CRADDOCK, I. ; LEENDERTZ, J. ; PREECE, A. ; BENJAMIN, R.: Experimental and clinical results of breast cancer detection using UWB microwave radar. In: *Proc. APS* (2008)

[26] KLEMM, M. ; CRADDOCK, I. ; LEENDERTZ, J. ; PREECE, A. ; BENJAMIN, R.: Clinical trials of a UWB imaging radar for breast cancer. In: *Proc. EuCAP* (2010)

[27] KLEMM, M. ; CRADDOCK, I. J. ; LEENDERTZ, J.A. ; PREECE, A. ; BENJAMIN, R.: Radar-based breast cancer detection using a hemispherical antenna array-Experimental results. In: *IEEE Trans. Antennas Propagat.* 57 (2009), Nr. 6, S. 1692 –1704

[28] KLEMM, M. ; LEENDERTZ, J. ; GIBBINS, D. ; CRADDOCK, I. ; PREECE, A. ; BENJAMIN, R.: Microwave radar-based differntial breast cancer imaging: imaging in homogeneous breast phantoms and low contrast scenarios. In: *IEEE Trans. Antennas Propag.* 58 (2010), Nr. 7, S. 2337 –2344

[29] L. GUO, A. M. A.: Optimization-Based Confocal Microwave Imaging in Medical Applications. In: *IEEE Trans. on Antennas Propag.* 63 (2015), S. 3531–3539

[30] LAZEBNIK, M. ; POPOVIC, D. ; MCCARTNEY, L. ; WATKINS, C. B. ; LINDSTROM, M. J. ; HARTER, J. ; SEWALL, S. ; OGILVIE, T. ; MAGLIOCCO, A. ; BRESLIN, T.M. ; TEMPLE, W. ; MEW, D. ; BOOSKE, J.H. ; OKONIEWSKI, M. ; ; HAGNESS, S.C.: A large-scale study of the ultrawideband microwave dielectric properties of normal, benign and malignant breast tissues obtained from cancer surgeries. In: *Phys. Med. and Biol.* 52 (2007), S. 6093–6115

[31] LI, X. ; BOND, E. J. ; VEEN, B. D. V. ; HAGNESS, S. C.: An overview of ultra-wideband microwave imaging via space-time beamforming for early-stage breast-cancer detection. In: *IEEE Antennas Propag. Mag.* 47 (2005), S. 19–34

[32] LI, X. ; JALILVAND, M. ; SIT, L. ; ZWICK, T: A Compact double-layer on-body matched Bowtie antenna for medical diagnostics. In: *IEEE Trans. on Antennas Propag.* 62 (2014), Nr. 4, S. 1808–1816

[33] LI, X. ; JALILVAND, M. ; ZWIRELLO, L. ; ZWICK, T.: Array configurations of a UWB near field imaging system for the detection of water accumulation in human body. In: *Proc. European Radar Conference EuRAD* (2011)

[34] LI, X. ; SIT, Y. ; ZWIRELLO, L. ; JALILVAND, M. ; ZWICK, T.: An E-field probe-based near-field measurement system for on- and in-body antennas. In: *Proc. IEEE EuMW* (2012)

[35] LI, X. ; SIT, Y. L. ; ZWIRELLO, L. ; ZWICK, T.: A miniaturized UWB stepped-slot antenna for medical diagnostic imaging. In: *Microwave and Optical lett.* 55 (2013), Nr. 1, S. 105–109

[36] M. AHADI, M. Saripan W. H. M. Isa I. M. Isa: Square monopole antenna for microwave imaging, design and characterisation. In: *IET Microw. Antennas Propag.* 9 (2015), S. 49–57

[37] MALLORQUI, J. J. ; JOACHIMOWICZ, N. ; BROQUETAS, A. ; BOLOMEY, J. C.: Quantitative images of large biological bodies in microwave tomography by using numerical and real data. In: *Electronics Letters* 32 (1996), S. 2138 – 2140

[38] MEANEY, P. M. ; FANNING, M. W. ; RAYNOLDS, T. ; FOX, C. J. ; FANG, Q. Q. ; KOGEL, C. A. ; POPLACK, S. P. ; PAULSEN, K. D.: Initial clinical experience with microwave breast imaging in women with normal mammography. In: *Acad. Radiol.* 14 (2007), S. 207–218

[39] MEANEY, P. M. ; GOODWIN, D. ; GOLNABI, A. H. ; ZHOU, T. ; PALLONE, M. ; GEIMER, S. D. ; BURKE, G. ; PAULSEN, K. D.: Clinical microwave tomographic imaging of the calcaneus: A first-in-human case study of two subjects. In: *IEEE Trans. Biomed. Eng.* 59 (2012), S. 3304–3313

[40] MEANEY, P. M. ; PAULSEN, K. D. ; HARTOV, A. ; CRANE, R. K.: An active microwave imaging system for reconstruction of 2-D electrical property distributions. In: *IEEE Trans. Biomed. Eng.* 42 (1995), Nr. 10, S. 1017–1027

[41] MIZUSHINA, S. ; OHBA, H. ; ABE, K. ; MIZOSHIRI, S. ; SUGIURA, T.: Recent trends in medical microwave radiometry. In: *IEIC Trans. Commun. Eng.* E78-B (1995), S. 789–798

[42] MOBASHSHER, A. T. ; ABBOSH, A. M.: Wideband unidirectional antenna for head imaging system. In: *Proc. IEEE APSURSI* (2013)

[43] MOBASHSHER, A. T. ; ABBOSH, A. M.: Compact Three-dimensional Slot-Loaded Folded Dipole Antenna with Unidirectional Radiation and Low Impulse Distortion for Head Imaging Applications. In: *Proc. IEEE APSURSI* (2014)

[44] MOBASHSHER, A. T. ; ABBOSH, A. M.: Near-field time-domain characterisation of wideband antennas. In: *Electronics Letters* 51 (2015), S. 2076–2078

[45] MOHAMMED, B. J. ; ABBOSH, A. M. ; MUSTAFA, S. ; IRELAND, D.: Microwave system for head imaging. In: *IEEE Trans. Instrum. Meas.* 63 (2014), S. 117–123

[46] MOJABI, P. ; LOVETRI, J.: Microwave Biomedical Imaging Using the Multiplicative Regularized Gauss–Newton Inversion. In: *IEEE Anten. and Wireless Propag. lett.* 8 (2009), S. 645 – 648

[47] MUIR, K. W. ; BUCHAN, A. ; KUMMER, R. von ; ROTHER, J. ; BARON, J. C.: Imaging of acute stroke. In: *Lancet Neurology* 5 (2006), S. 755–768

[48] MUSTAFA, S. ; MOHAMMED, B. ; ABBOSH, A.: Novel Preprocessing Techniques for Accurate Microwave Imaging of Human Brain. In: *IEEE Anten. and Wireless Propag. lett.* 12 (2013), S. 460–463

[49] NIKOLOVA, N.: Microwave imaging for breast cancer. In: *IEEE Microwave magazine* 12 (2011), Dec., Nr. 7, S. 78–94

[50] OBEID, D. ; SADEK, S. ; ZAHARIA, G. ; ZEIN, G. E.: Multitunable microwave system for touchless heartbeat detection and heart rate variability extraction. In: *Microw. Opt. Tech. Lett.* 52 (2010), S. 192–198

[51] O'HALLORAN, M. ; JONES, E. ; GLAVIN, M.: Quasi-multistatic MIST beamforming for the early detection of breast cancer. In: *IEEE Trans. Biomed. Imaging* 57 (2010), Nr. 4, S. 830 –840

[52] OSKOOI, A. F. ; ROUNDY, D. ; IBANESCU, M. ; BERMEL, P. ; JOANNOPOULOS, J. D. ; JOHNSON, S. G.: MEEP: A flexible free-software package for electromagnetic simulations by the FDTD method. In: *Computer Physics Communications* 181 (2010), Jul., Nr. 6, S. 1692 –1704

[53] OSTADRAHIMI, M. ; MOJABI, P. ; GILMORE, C. ; ZAKARIA, A. ; NOGHANIAN, S. ; PISTORIUS, S. ; LOVETRI, J.: Analysis of Incident Field Modeling and Incident/Scattered Field Calibration Techniques in Microwave Tomography. In: *IEEE Anten. and Wireless Propag. lett.* 10 (2011), S. 900–903

[54] OSTADRAHIMI, M. ; MOJABI, P. ; NOGHANIAN, S. ; SHAFAI, L. ; PISTORIUS, S. ; LOVETRI, J.: A Novel Microwave Tomography System Based on the Scattering Probe Technique. In: *IEEE Transactions on Instrumentation and Measurement* 61 (2012), S. 379–390

[55] PARK, S. ; KARPIOUK, A. B. ; AGLYAMOV, S. R. ; EMELIANOV, S. Y.: Adaptive beamforming for photoacoustic imaging. In: *Optical lett.* 33 (2008), Nr. 12, S. 1291–1293

[56] PERSSON, M. ; FHAGER, A. ; TREFNÃ¡, H. D. ; YU, Y. ; MCKELVEY, T. ; PEGENIUS, G. ; KARLSSON, J. ; ELAM, M.: Microwave-Based stroke diagnosis making global prehospital thrombolytic treatment possible. In: *IEEE Trans. Biomed. Eng.* 61 (2014), S. 2806–2817

[57] POZAR, D. M.: Microwave Engineering. In: *Wiley* (2004)

[58] Q. FANG, P. M. M. ; PAULSEN, K. D.: Microwave image reconstruction of tissue property dispersion characteristics utilizing multiple-frequency information. In: *IEEE Trans. Microwave Theory Tech.* 52 (2004), S. 1866–1875

[59] REZAEIEH, S. A. ; ZAMANI, A. ; ABBOSH, A. M.: 3-D Wideband Antenna for Head-Imaging System with Performance Verification in Brain Tumor Detection. In: *IEEE Anten. and Wireless Propag. lett.* 14 (2015), S. 910–914

[60] ROSAMOND, W. ; FLEGAL, K. ; FRIDAY, G.: Heart disease and stroke statisticsâ2007 update: a report from the American Heart Association Statistics Committee and Stroke Statistics Subcommittee. In: *Circulation* 115 (2007), S. 69–171

[61] S. Y. SEMENOV, D. R. C.: Microwave Tomography for Brain Imaging: Feasibility Assessment for Stroke Detection. In: *International Journal of Antennas and Propag.* (2008)

[62] SACHSE, F. B. ; WERNER, C. ; MÃ¼LLER, M. ; MEYER-WAARDEN, K.: Segmentation and tissue classification of the visible man dataset using the computer tomographic scans and the thin-section photo. In: *Proc. 1st Users Conf. National Library of Medicine* 28 (1996), S. 125–126

[63] SADIKU, M. N. O.: Numerical Techniques in Electromagnetics with MATLAB. In: *CRC Press* (2009)

[64] SALVADOR, S. M. ; FEAR, E. C. ; OKONIEWSKI, M. ; MATYAS, J. R.: Exploring joint tissues with microwave imaging. In: *IEEE Trans. Microw. Theory Tech.* 58 (2010), S. 2307–2313

[65] SCAPATICCI, R. ; DONATO, L. D. ; CATAPANO, I. ; CROCCO, L.: A feasibility study on microwave imaging for brain stroke monitoring. In: *IEEE Trans. Instrum. Meas.* 40 (2012), S. 305–324

[66] SCHWARZ, U. ; THIEL, F. ; SEIFERT, F. ; STEPHAN, R. ; HEIN, M.: Ultra-wideband antennas for combined magnetic resonance imaging and UWB radar applications. In: *IEEE MTT-s international* (2009)

[67] SEMENOV, S. Y.: Microwave tomography: review of the progress towards clinical applications. In: *Philosoph-ical Transactions* (2009)

[68] SEMENOV, S. Y. ; BULYSHEV, A. E. ; ABUBAKAR, A. ; POSUKH, V. G. ; SIZOV, Y. E. ; SOUVOROV, A. E. ; BERG, P. M. d. ; WILLIAMS, T. C.: Microwave-tomographic imaging of the high dielectric-contrast objects using different image-reconstruction approaches. In: *IEEE Trans. Microwave Theory Tech.* 53 (2005), S. 2284–2294

[69] SEMENOV, S. Y. ; BULYSHEV, A. E. ; POSUKH, V. G. ; SIZOV, Y. E. ; WILLIAMS, T. C.: Microwave tomography for detection/imaging of myocardial infarction. I. Excised canine hearts. In: *Ann. Biomed. Eng.* 31 (2003), S. 262–270

[70] SEMENOV, S. Y. ; BULYSHEV, A. E. ; SOUVOROV, A. E. ; SVENSON, R. H. ; SIZOV, Y. E. ; VORISOV, V. Y. ; POSUKH, V. G. ; KOZLOV, I. M. ; NAZAROV, A. G. ; TATSIS, G. P.: Microwave tomography: theoretical and experimental investigation of the iteration reconstruction algorithm. In: *IEEE Trans. on Microwave Theory and Techniques* 46 (1998), S. 133–141

[71] SILL, J. M. ; FEAR, E. C.: Tissue sensing adaptive radar for breast cancer detectionâExperimental investigation of simple tumor models. In: *IEEE Trans. Microw. Theory Tech.* 53 (2005), S. 3312–3319

[72] SON, S. ; SIMONOV, N. ; KIM, H. ; LEE, J. ; JEON, S.: Preclinical Prototype Development of a Microwave Tomography System for Breast Cancer Detection. In: *ETRI Journal* 32 (2010), S. 901–910

[73] T. YIN, C. Reyes-Aldasoro F. H. A. F. H. Ali: A Robust and Artifact Resistant Algorithm of Ultrawideband Imaging System for Breast Cancer Detection. In: *IEEE Trans. Biomed. Eng.* 62 (2015), S. 1514–1525

[74] WU, J. ; NYBORG, W.: Emerging therapeutic ultrasound. In: *World Scienctific* (2006), S. 179–280

[75] YANG, F. ; CHEN, Y. ; WANG, R. ; ZHANG, Q.: Super-resolution microwave imaging: Time-domain tomography using highly accurate evolutionary optimization method. In: *Proc. EuCAP* (2015)

[76] YU, C. ; YUAN, M. ; STANG, J. ; BRESSLOUR, E. ; GEORGE, R. T. ; YBARRA, G. A. ; JOINES, W. T. ; LIU, Q. H.: Active microwave imaging II: 3-D system prototype and image reconstruction from experimental data. In: *IEEE Trans. Microw. Theory Tech.* 56 (2008), Nr. 4, S. 991–1000

[77] YUN, X. ; FEAR, E. C. ; JOHNSTON, R. H.: Compact antenna for radar-based breast cancer detection. In: *IEEE Trans. Antennas Propag.* 53 (2005), S. 2374–2380

[78] ZAEYTIJD, J. D. ; FRANCHOIS, A. ; EYRAUD, C. ; GEFFRIN, J. M.: Full-wave three-dimentional microwave imaging with a regularized Gauss-Newton method- Theory and experiment. In: *IEEE Trans. Antennas Propagat.* 55 (2007), S. 3279–3292

[79] Zakrzewski, M. ; Raittinen, H. ; Vanhala, J.: Comparison of center estimation algorithms for heart and respiration monitoring with microwave doppler radar. In: *IEEE Sensors J.* 12 (2012), S. 627–634

[80] Zhu, X. Z. ; Zhao, Z. Q. ; Yang, K. ; Nie, Z. P. ; Liu, Q. H.: A prototype system of microwave induced thermo-acoustic tomography for breast tumor. In: *Proc. Annu. Int. Conf. Eng. Med. Biol. Soc.* 56 (2012), S. 464–467

[81] Zhurbenko, V. ; Rubaek, T. ; Krozer, V. ; Meincke, P.: Design and realisation of a microwave three-dimensional imaging system with application to breast-cancer detection. In: *IET Microwaves, Antennas Propag.* 4 (2010), S. 2200–2211

Own Publications

Journals

M. Jalilvand, X. Li, L. Zwirello and T. Zwick. Ultra wideband compact near-field imaging system for breast cancer detection, *IET Microwaves, Antennas Propagation*, 2015, Vol.9, pp. 1009 - 1014.

M. Jalilvand, X. Li, J. Kowalewski and T. Zwick. Broadband miniaturised bowtie antenna for 3D microwave tomography, *Electronics Letters*, 2014, Vol.50, pp. 244 - 246.

M. Jalilvand, Ch. Wu, J. Schmid and T. Zwick. Quantitative imaging of numerically realistic human head model using microwave tomography, *Electronics Letters*, 2014, Vol.50, pp. 255 - 256, *(distinguished as feature article)*.

X. Li, M. Jalilvand, L. Sit and T. Zwick. A Compact Double-Layer On-Body Matched Bowtie Antenna for Medical Diagnostics, *IEEE Transactions on Antennas and Propagation*, 2014, Vol.62, pp. 1808 - 1816.

Conferences

M. Jalilvand, C. Vasanelli, C. Wu, J. Kowalewski and T. Zwick. On the evaluation of a proposed bowtie antenna for microwave tomography, *Proc. EuCAP*, 2014.

M. Jalilvand, X. Li, T. Zwick, W. Wiesbeck and E. Pancera. Hemorrhagic stroke detection via UWB medical imaging, *Proc. EuCAP*, 2011.

M. Jalilvand, T. Zwick, W. Wiesbeck and E. Pancera. UWB synthetic aperture-based radar system for hemorrhagic head-stroke detection, *IEEE RadarCon (RADAR)*, 2011.

M. Jalilvand, X. Li and T. Zwick. A model approach to the analytical analysis of stroke detection using UWB radar, *Proc. EuCAP*, 2013.

M. Jalilvand, C. Vasanelli, J. Kowalewski and T. Zwick. Implementation of Antenna Array Systems for Medical Imaging, *Proc. Gemic*, 2014.

M. Jalilvand, E. Pancera, X. Li, T. Zwick and W. Wiesbeck. A sparse Synthetic Aperture-based UWB medical imaging system, *Proc. Gemic*, 2011.

X. Li, Y.L. Sit, L. Zwirello, M. Jalilvand and T. Zwick. An E-field probe based near-field measurement system for on- and in-body antennas, *Proc. EuMC*, 2012.

X. Li, M. Jalilvand, L. Zwirello and T. Zwick. Array configurations of a UWB near field imaging system for the detection of water accumulation in human body, *Proc. EuRAD*, 2011.

X. Li, M. Jalilvand, J. Yan, L. Zwirello and T. Zwick. A multiband slotted Bowtie antenna for stroke detection, *Proc. Ultra-Wideband*, 2012.

E. Pancera, X. Li, M. Jalilvand, T. Zwick and W. Wiesbeck. UWB medical diagnostic: in-body transmission modeling and applications, *Proc. Eucap*, 2011.

X. Li, J. Yan, M. Jalilvand and T. Zwick. A compact double-elliptical slot-antenna for medical applications, *Proc. Eucap*, 2012.

E. Pancera, H. Barbara, X. Li, M. Jalilvand and T. Zwick. UWB antennas optimization for in-body radiation, *Proc. Gemic*, 2011.

X. Li, L. Zwirello, M. Jalilvand and T. Zwick. Design and near-field characterization of a planar on-body UWB slot-antenna for stroke detection, *Proc. iWAT*, 2012.

X. Li, M. Jalilvand, L. Zwirello and T. Zwick. Synthetic aperture-based UWB imaging system for detection of urine accumulation in human bladder, *Proc. ICUWB*, 2011.

X. Li, M. Jalilvand, W. You, W. Wiesbeck and T. Zwick. An implantable stripline-fed slot antenna for biomedical applications, *Proc. IET Radar*, 2013.

Forschungsberichte aus dem Institut für Höchstfrequenztechnik und Elektronik (IHE) der Universität Karlsruhe (TH)
(ISSN 0942-2935)

Herausgeber: Prof. Dr.-Ing. Dr. h.c. Dr.-Ing. E.h. mult. Werner Wiesbeck

Band 1 Daniel Kähny
Modellierung und meßtechnische Verifikation polarimetrischer, mono- und bistatischer Radarsignaturen und deren Klassifizierung (1992)

Band 2 Eberhardt Heidrich
Theoretische und experimentelle Charakterisierung der polarimetrischen Strahlungs- und Streueigenschaften von Antennen (1992)

Band 3 Thomas Kürner
Charakterisierung digitaler Funksysteme mit einem breitbandigen Wellenausbreitungsmodell (1993)

Band 4 Jürgen Kehrbeck
Mikrowellen-Doppler-Sensor zur Geschwindigkeits- und Wegmessung – System-Modellierung und Verifikation (1993)

Band 5 Christian Bornkessel
Analyse und Optimierung der elektrodynamischen Eigenschaften von EMV-Absorberkammern durch numerische Feldberechnung (1994)

Band 6 Rainer Speck
Hochempfindliche Impedanzmessungen an Supraleiter / Festelektrolyt-Kontakten (1994)

Band 7 Edward Pillai
Derivation of Equivalent Circuits for Multilayer PCB and Chip Package Discontinuities Using Full Wave Models (1995)

Band 8 Dieter J. Cichon
Strahlenoptische Modellierung der Wellenausbreitung in urbanen Mikro- und Pikofunkzellen (1994)

Band 9 Gerd Gottwald
Numerische Analyse konformer Streifenleitungsantennen in mehrlagigen Zylindern mittels der Spektralbereichsmethode (1995)

Band 10 Norbert Geng
Modellierung der Ausbreitung elektromagnetischer Wellen in Funksystemen durch Lösung der parabolischen Approximation der Helmholtz-Gleichung (1996)

Band 11 Torsten C. Becker
Verfahren und Kriterien zur Planung von Gleichwellennetzen für den Digitalen Hörrundfunk DAB (Digital Audio Broadcasting) (1996)

Band 12 Friedhelm Rostan
Dual polarisierte Microstrip-Patch-Arrays für zukünftige satellitengestützte SAR-Systeme (1996)

Band 13 Markus Demmler
Vektorkorrigiertes Großsignal-Meßsystem zur nichtlinearen Charakterisierung von Mikrowellentransistoren (1996)

Band 14 Andreas Froese
Elektrochemisches Phasengrenzverhalten von Supraleitern (1996)

Band 15 Jürgen v. Hagen
Wide Band Electromagnetic Aperture Coupling to a Cavity: An Integral Representation Based Model (1997)

Band 16 Ralf Pötzschke
Nanostrukturierung von Festkörperflächen durch elektrochemische Metallphasenbildung (1998)

Band 17 Jean Parlebas
Numerische Berechnung mehrlagiger dualer planarer Antennen mit koplanarer Speisung (1998)

Band 18 Frank Demmerle
Bikonische Antenne mit mehrmodiger Anregung für den räumlichen Mehrfachzugriff (SDMA) (1998)

Band 19 Eckard Steiger
Modellierung der Ausbreitung in extrakorporalen Therapien eingesetzter Ultraschallimpulse hoher Intensität (1998)

Band 20 Frederik Küchen
Auf Wellenausbreitungsmodellen basierende Planung terrestrischer COFDM-Gleichwellennetze für den mobilen Empfang (1998)

Band 21 Klaus Schmitt
Dreidimensionale, interferometrische Radarverfahren im Nahbereich und ihre meßtechnische Verifikation (1998)

Band 22 Frederik Küchen, Torsten C. Becker, Werner Wiesbeck
Grundlagen und Anwendungen von Planungswerkzeugen für den digitalen terrestrischen Rundfunk (1999)

Band 23 Thomas Zwick
Die Modellierung von richtungsaufgelösten Mehrwegegebäudefunkkanälen durch markierte Poisson-Prozesse (2000)

Band 24 Dirk Didascalou
Ray-Optical Wave Propagation Modelling in Arbitrarily Shaped Tunnels (2000)

Band 25 Hans Rudolf
Increase of Information by Polarimetric Radar Systems (2000)

Band 26 Martin Döttling
Strahlenoptisches Wellenausbreitungsmodell und Systemstudien für den Satellitenmobilfunk (2000)

Band 27 Jens Haala
Analyse von Mikrowellenheizprozessen mittels selbstkonsistenter finiter Integrationsverfahren (2000)

Band 28 Eberhard Gschwendtner
Breitbandige Multifunktionsantennen für den konformen Einbau in Kraftfahrzeuge (2001)

Band 29 Dietmar Löffler
Breitbandige, zylinderkonforme Streifenleitungsantennen für den Einsatz in Kommunikation und Sensorik (2001)

Band 30 Xuemin Huang
Automatic Cell Planning for Mobile Network Design: Optimization Models and Algorithms (2001)

Band 31 Martin Fritzsche
Anwendung von Verfahren der Mustererkennung zur Detektion von Landminen mit Georadaren (2001)

Band 32 Siegfried Ginter
Selbstkonsistente Modellierung der Erhitzung von biologischem Gewebe durch hochintensiven Ultraschall (2002)

Band 33 Young Jin Park
Applications of Photonic Bandgap Structures with Arbitrary Surface Impedance to Luneburg Lenses for Automotive Radar (2002)

Band 34 Alexander Herschlein
Entwicklung numerischer Verfahren zur Feldberechnung konformer Antennen auf Oberflächen höherer Ordnung (2002)

Band 35 Ralph Schertlen
Mikrowellenprozessierung nanotechnologischer Strukturen am Beispiel von Zeolithen (2002)

Band 36 Jürgen von Hagen
Numerical Algorithms for the Solution of Linear Systems of Equations Arising in Computational Electromagnetics (2002)

Band 37 Ying Zhang
Artificial Perfect Magnetic Conductor and its Application to Antennas (2003)

Band 38 Thomas M. Schäfer
Experimentelle und simulative Analyse der Funkwellenausbreitung in Kliniken (2003)

Band 39 Christian Fischer
Multistatisches Radar zur Lokalisierung von Objekten im Boden (2003)

Band 40 Yan C. Venot
Entwicklung und Integration eines Nahbereichsradarsensorsystems bei 76,5 GHz (2004)

Band 41 Christian Waldschmidt
Systemtheoretische und experimentelle Charakterisierung integrierbarer Antennenarrays (2004)

Band 42 Marwan Younis
Digital Beam-Forming for high Resolution Wide Swath Real and Synthetic Aperture Radar (2004)

Band 43 Jürgen Maurer
Strahlenoptisches Kanalmodell für die Fahrzeug-Fahrzeug-Funkkommunikation (2005)

Band 44 Florian Pivit
Multiband-Aperturantennen für Basisstationsanwendungen in rekonfigurierbaren Mobilfunksystemen (2005)

Band 45 Sergey Sevskiy
Multidirektionale logarithmisch-periodische Indoor-Basisstationsantennen (2006)

Band 46 Martin Fritz
Entwurf einer breitbandigen Leistungsendstufe für den Mobilfunk in Low Temperature Cofired Ceramic (2006)

Band 47 Christiane Kuhnert
Systemanalyse von Mehrantennen-Frontends (MIMO) (2006)

Band 48 Marco Liebler
Modellierung der dynamischen Wechselwirkungen von hoch-intensiven Ultraschallfeldern mit Kavitationsblasen (2006)

Band 49 Thomas Dreyer
Systemmodellierung piezoelektrischer Sender zur Erzeugung hochintensiver Ultraschallimpulse für die medizinische Therapie (2006)

Band 50 Stephan Schulteis
Integration von Mehrantennensystemen in kleine mobile Geräte für multimediale Anwendungen (2007)

Band 51 Werner Sörgel
Charakterisierung von Antennen für die Ultra-Wideband-Technik (2007)

Band 52 Reiner Lenz
Hochpräzise, kalibrierte Transponder und Bodenempfänger für satellitengestützte SAR-Missionen (2007)

Band 53 Christoph Schwörer
Monolithisch integrierte HEMT-basierende Frequenzvervielfacher und Mischer oberhalb 100 GHz (2008)

Band 54 Karin Schuler
Intelligente Antennensysteme für Kraftfahrzeug-Nahbereichs-Radar-Sensorik (2007)

Band 55 Christian Römer
Slotted waveguide structures in phased array antennas (2008)

Fortführung als „Karlsruher Forschungsberichte aus dem Institut für Hochfrequenztechnik und Elektronik bei KIT Scientific Publishing (ISSN 1868-4696)

Karlsruher Forschungsberichte aus dem Institut für Hochfrequenztechnik und Elektronik
(ISSN 1868-4696)

Herausgeber: Prof. Dr.-Ing. Thomas Zwick

Band 55 Sandra Knörzer
Funkkanalmodellierung für OFDM-Kommunikationssysteme bei Hochgeschwindigkeitszügen (2009)
ISBN 978-3-86644-361-7

Band 56 Thomas Fügen
Richtungsaufgelöste Kanalmodellierung und Systemstudien für Mehrantennensysteme in urbanen Gebieten (2009)
ISBN 978-3-86644-420-1

Band 57 Elena Pancera
Strategies for Time Domain Characterization of UWB Components and Systems (2009)
ISBN 978-3-86644-417-1

Band 58 Jens Timmermann
Systemanalyse und Optimierung der Ultrabreitband-Übertragung (2010)
ISBN 978-3-86644-460-7

Band 59 Juan Pontes
Analysis and Design of Multiple Element Antennas for Urban Communication (2010)
ISBN 978-3-86644-513-0

Band 60 Andreas Lambrecht
True-Time-Delay Beamforming für ultrabreitbandige Systeme hoher Leistung (2010)
ISBN 978-3-86644-522-2

Band 61 Grzegorz Adamiuk
Methoden zur Realisierung von dual-orthogonal, linear polarisierten Antennen für die UWB-Technik (2010)
ISBN 978-3-86644-573-4

Band 62 Jutta Kühn
AlGaN/GaN-HEMT Power Amplifiers with Optimized Power-Added Efficiency for X-Band Applications (2011)
ISBN 978-3-86644-615-1

Band 63 Małgorzata Janson
Hybride Funkkanalmodellierung für ultrabreitbandige MIMO-Systeme (2011)
ISBN 978-3-86644-639-7

Band 64 Mario Pauli
Dekontaminierung verseuchter Böden durch Mikrowellenheizung (2011)
ISBN 978-3-86644-696-0

Band 65 Thorsten Kayser
Feldtheoretische Modellierung der Materialprozessierung mit Mikrowellen im Durchlaufbetrieb (2011)
ISBN 978-3-86644-719-6

Band 66 Christian Andreas Sturm
Gemeinsame Realisierung von Radar-Sensorik und Funkkommunikation mit OFDM-Signalen (2012)
ISBN 978-3-86644-879-7

Band 67 Huaming Wu
Motion Compensation for Near-Range Synthetic Aperture Radar Applications (2012)
ISBN 978-3-86644-906-0

Band 68 Friederike Brendel
Millimeter-Wave Radio-over-Fiber Links based on Mode-Locked Laser Diodes (2013)
ISBN 978-3-86644-986-2

Band 69 Lars Reichardt
Methodik für den Entwurf von kapazitätsoptimierten Mehrantennensystemen am Fahrzeug (2013)
ISBN 978-3-7315-0047-6

Band 70 Stefan Beer
Methoden und Techniken zur Integration von 122 GHz Antennen in miniaturisierte Radarsensoren (2013)
ISBN 978-3-7315-0051-3

Band 71 Łukasz Zwirełło
Realization Limits of Impulse-Radio UWB Indoor Localization Systems (2013)
ISBN 978-3-7315-0114-5

Band 72 Xuyang Li
Body Matched Antennas for Microwave Medical Applications (2014)
ISBN 978-3-7315-0147-3

Band 73 Sebastian Diebold
Transistor- und Leitungsmodellierung zum Entwurf von monolithisch integrierten Leistungsverstärkern für den hohen Millimeterwellen-Frequenzbereich (2014)
ISBN 978-3-7315-0161-9

Band 74 Christian Rusch
Integrierte, planare Leckwellenantennen für 3D-Millimeterwellen-Radarsysteme basierend auf dem holografischen Prinzip (2014)
ISBN 978-3-7315-0234-0

Band 75 Marlene Harter
Dreidimensional bildgebendes Radarsystem mit digitaler Strahlformung für industrielle Anwendungen (2014)
ISBN 978-3-7315-0249-4

Band 76 Michael A. Baldauf
Abhängigkeit der Exposition von der Zellgröße beim Mobilfunk unter Gewährleistung der Versorgung (2015)
ISBN 978-3-7315-0308-8

Band 77 Alicja Ossowska
Highly Resolved Synthetic Aperture Radar with Beam Steering (2015)
ISBN 978-3-7315-0315-6

Band 78 Małgorzata Dominika Brzeska
RF Modelling and Characterization of Tyre Pressure Sensors and Vehicle Access Systems (2015)
ISBN 978-3-7315-0348-4

Band 79 Ulrich Lewark
Aktive Frequenzvervielfacher zur Signalerzeugung im Millimeter- und Submillimeterwellen Frequenzbereich (2015)
ISBN 978-3-7315-0354-5

Band 80 Kai-Philipp Walter Pahl
Distributed Transformers for Broadband Monolithic Millimeter-Wave Integrated Power Amplifiers (2015)
ISBN 978-3-7315-0409-2

Band 81 Serdal Ayhan
Hochgenaue radarbasierte Abstandsmessung mit geführter Wellenausbreitung (2016)
ISBN 978-3-7315-0433-7

Band 82 Yoke Leen Sit
MIMO OFDM Radar-Communication System with Mutual Interference Cancellation (2017)
ISBN 978-3-7315-0599-0

Band 83 Steffen Scherr
FMCW-Radarsignalverarbeitung zur Entfernungsmessung mit hoher Genauigkeit (2017)
ISBN 978-3-7315-0607-2

Band 84 Tom Schipper
Modellbasierte Analyse des Interferenzverhaltens von Kfz-Radaren (2017)
ISBN 978-3-7315-0639-3

Band 85 Malyhe Jalilvand
Application-Specific Broadband Antennas for Microwave Medical Imaging (2017)
ISBN 978-3-7315-0664-5

Die Bände sind unter www.ksp.kit.edu als PDF frei verfügbar oder als Druckausgabe bestellbar.